Weight Loss
&
Healthy Eating

Other books available include:

Motivation, Achievement & Challenges

Understanding & Building Confidence

Managing Stress & Preventing Depression

Real Benefits of Exercise

How to Sleep Better!

Please make a donation if you can

TEXT: BOOK32£5

To: 70070

Or an online donation via:

www.justgiving.com/healthbooks

www.cymhealth.org

THANK YOU!

Weight Loss
&
Healthy Eating

by

Charlie Wardle

Climb Your Mountain

Copyright © Charlie Wardle 2015

The right of Charlie Wardle to be identified as the author of this work has been asserted in accordance with the Copyright, Designs & Patents Act 1988.

All rights reserved. No part of this book may be reproduced, stored in a retrieval system, or transmitted in any form or by any means, electronic, electrostatic, magnetic tape, mechanical, photocopying, recording or otherwise, without the written permission of the copyright holder.

Published under licence by Brown Dog Books and

The Self Publishing Partnership

7 Green Park Station, Bath BA1 1JB

www.selfpublishingpartnership.co.uk

ISBN book: 978-1-903056-97-4

ISBN e-book: 978-1-903056-98-1

Cover design by Kevin Rylands

Printed and bound by CPI Group (UK) Ltd, Croydon CR0 4YY

Contents

About the author 8

Introduction 9
    Questionnaires 12

Part 1 – Weight loss 17

Introduction 27

Being overweight – the issues 18
- *Physical health* 18
- *Emotional health* 26
- *It's not all about your weight and weight loss* 30

Why are so many people overweight? 32
- *We eat too much* 32
- *We eat the wrong food types* 33
- *Sugar addiction* 34
- *Lack of exercise and activity* 36
- *Stress, depression and anxiety* 37
- *Habit, choices and excuses* 37
- *Lack of accountability and personal responsibility* 38
- *Diets – fads and fiction* 39
- *Poor sleep* 41
- *Boredom* 41
- *Obesity becoming normalised in society* 42

Losing weight 44
- *Sensible approach* 44
- *The weight-loss equation (calories)* 45

- Motivation, reasons and goals   45
- The right support   46
- Be careful of the common pitfalls   47
- Eating out, treats, celebrations and holidays   48
- Cutting out the sugar!   49
- Grow your own fruit and vegetables   50
- Exercise and activity   51
- Good food types   52
- The right times to eat   53
- Portion sizes   54
- Weight loss for children   55
- Make it a lifestyle   56

Part 2 – Healthy eating   57

Introduction   57

Understanding Food   58
- Understanding calories   58
- Understanding fats   61
- Understanding salt   65
- Understanding carbohydrates   67
- Understanding proteins   69
- Understanding fibre   69
- Understanding vitamins and minerals   72
- Vegetables and salads   76
- Understanding processed foods   78

Other Factors   80
- The benefits of water and hydration   80
- Alcohol   80
- Food and mood   82

- *Preventing illness 83*
- *Cooking healthily 84*
- *Food allergies and intolerances 85*

Case Study 87

Suggested Nutrition Plan 89

Summary and Moving Forward 91

The CYM Weight Loss Challenge 94

About the 'Climb Your Mountain' Charity 95

About the author

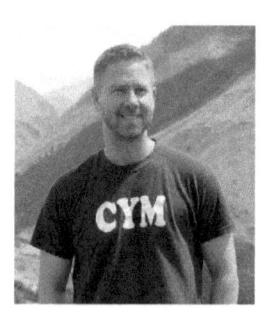

Charlie Wardle founded the Climb Your Mountain (CYM) charity in 2008 with the objective of helping as many people as possible to climb the personal mountain they may face in their life for whatever reason. CYM provides a wide range of both educational and physical activity opportunities so that people can help themselves to a healthier and happier life. Previously, Charlie had a successful finance, accounting and marketing career with a number of large blue-chip companies. He is a qualified Chartered Accountant (ACA) and has an MBA from Cranfield School of Management. His passion is health, wellbeing and fitness.

The education and learning side, called CYM Health, offers a range of free health and wellbeing books, courses, workshops, videos, talks and advice which are written, delivered and presented by Charlie. He has spent the last few years researching, reading, thinking, discussing and meeting with hundreds of people in order to build up the knowledge and experience that is then offered to others.

Please read the section at the end of this book to find out more about the Climb Your Mountain (CYM) charity and also please visit the website www.climbyourmountain.org for an online video workshop focusing on this book. Plus make sure you read the other health and wellbeing books in this series.

Introduction

There is absolutely no doubt that more and more people are becoming overweight and many of these are becoming obese. There is also absolutely no doubt that being overweight and obese is unhealthy and in most cases will lead to a wide range of physical, mental and emotional health issues. It is a real concern yet it is also preventable. This book aims to provide information and knowledge for people to give them a better chance of losing weight and eating more healthily so that they can benefit from being healthier and happier as a result.

There are many reasons why people are becoming more and more overweight and it is important to look at all of these and try to work out what factors apply or might apply to you. You may be aware of many of these already, but perhaps you are not so aware of all the effects and consequences and how by being more knowledgeable, making better choices, changing habits and prioritising more your own health, significant benefits can be gained.

One of the major factors leading to excess weight and obesity is what we eat and drink. The second section of the book looks at healthy eating and how with greater understanding and knowledge we will be better placed to make more of the right choices when it comes to our health.

In the modern, developed, westernised world we live in there are so many choices and temptations that often lead us to eat and drink the wrong things in terms of our health. It is far easier to eat 'fast food', to buy a takeaway, to go for ready meals and other conveniently made processed foods. So much of the food available is addictive, with high sugar content, and portion sizes continue to increase far more than is needed. The easy choices when it comes to food and drink are nearly always the unhealthy choices. However, it is only really by understanding the effects and consequences to our health that we are likely to change and begin to make more of the right choices.

With lots of pressures, stress, demands, lack of time, convenience foods, strong marketing by food manufacturers and retailers, addictive foods, bargains on offer and many more factors it is not surprising that there has been such an increase in people being overweight in the last few decades. The responsibility, though, does always come down to the individual and although there are many reasons and factors, ultimately it is the individual who puts the food and drink in their own mouth.

Physical conditions and illness are rapidly increasing due to people being overweight and obese and the risks of serious disease increases considerably the more overweight you are. Many mental and emotional health problems are a cause or effect of being overweight and this is also a growing problem. So the message of the book is really that if you wish to be healthier and happier then understand the factors, become more knowledgeable, make more of an effort and make more of the healthy choices. It can work and it does work and the results and rewards are worth it. Plus you can not only lead a healthier and happier life for yourself but also become an inspiration for others too!

Introduction

A few interesting statistics

(From 'The Health and Social Care Information Centre' for the NHS published in 2013)

- The proportion of adults with a normal BMI decreased between 1993 and 2011 from 41% to 34% among men and from 50% to 39% among women.

- There was a marked increase in the proportion of adults that were obese from 13% in 1993 to 24% in 2011 for men and from 16% to 26% for women.

- 24% of men and 29% of women consumed the recommended five or more portions of fruit and vegetables daily in 2011 (27% of adults aged 16 and over).

- Of 5-15 year old boys, 16% consumed 5 or more portions of fruit and vegetables daily in 2011. For girls aged 5-15 the figure was 20%.

- Mean consumption of fruit and vegetables for children aged 11 to 18 years was 3.0 portions per day for boys and 2.8 portions per day for girls. 11% of boys and 8% of girls in this age group met the "5-a-day" recommendation.

- More than four in five children regarded their diet as healthy with most saying it was quite healthy (70% of boys and 72% of girls) rather than very healthy (13% of both boys and girls). Only 1% thought that their diet was very unhealthy.

- In 2011, obese adults (aged 16 and over) were more likely to have high blood pressure than those in the normal weight group. High blood pressure was recorded in 53% of men and 44% of women in the obese group and in 16% of men and 14% of women in the normal weight group.

Questionnaires

Before writing the book I sent out a questionnaire to a mix of people (young and old, male and female, overweight and good weight, etc.) and asked them the following four questions related to weight and healthy eating. Over the next few pages is a selection of real answers from real people, which I felt was representative of the general population.

What are the main reasons why you do not eat healthily?

- *When I'm in a rush / need a sugar hit / laziness.*

- *It used to be bad habits, laziness and just a lack of inspiration some days.*

- *Fresh food doesn't last as long. It's easier to get takeaway when you have been to work all day and don't feel like cooking. Healthy food doesn't always looks as appetising.*

- *Lack of time, is easier to grab something on the run.*

- *I live alone and lack motivation to home cook for just me.*

- *I'm a very busy girl with work, I sometimes forget to eat, then need to eat something straight away, so go for an easy option – call me a binge eater!*

- *I have a sweet tooth and love chocolate and cakes.*

- *If I feel down in the dumps or low about something I tend to eat more chocolate or sweet things.*

- *If I'm eating out I treat myself and have whatever I fancy.*

- *Too lazy to cook.*

- *Hassle of going to supermarkets, live on my own, fresh fruit and vegetables do not last very long, sugar addiction and cravings.*

What advice would you give to someone who is overweight and why?

- *I would advise a healthier diet due to the health issues of obesity/being overweight. E.g. the greater risk of heart disease, diabetes, arthritis and low self-esteem. I would oppose any 'fad' diets and suggest a healthy balanced diet with sensible portions. I would also suggest sensible exercise. Set yourself a realistic regime that can be attained over a period of time, not one that's a quick fix.*

- *Fix your low self-esteem and lack of self-worth issues and the rest will follow. It really does boil down to that even though it is not that simple to do!*

- *I would advise them to download the fitnesspal app and try calorie counting their intake of food. I would advise this as it was the thing that worked for me. I have been overweight myself and after years of dieting (using slimming world/Atkins/Weight watchers) the only thing that worked was comparing the calorie intake to calories burned.*

- *Depends on the situation really??... are they happy as overweight? In which case there is little you can do other than scare them on health issues to change. E.g. Do they want children now or in their future?... in which case such excess weight may prevent that.*

- *If they don't want to be overweight and are unhappy with themselves, then I would encourage them to make the change to their lifestyle – yoyo dieting isn't the answer, they need to make positive changes to the choices they make every day from food selection to keeping active.*

- *Keep a food diary so you can see what you're consuming on a daily basis and what times of the day you fall into a bad habit so you can try and combat them with better habits.*

- *Find some form of exercise that you enjoy and like doing*

- *Eat lots of fresh fruit and vegetables and wholegrain foods. Learn to love them!*

- Clear your cupboards of bad food and avoid the aisle in the shops COMPLETELY. Or shop online, you have much more control of what you buy. Treat yourself occasionally too, maybe when you've achieved something new.

- The effort to lose weight and be healthier will be worth it! You will feel so much better, have more energy, be more confident, be happier and it does become easier to lead a healthier lifestyle.

What motivates you to eat healthily and/or lose weight?

- Being aware of the body's requirements, conscious of my body image (which once was very negative) but, more importantly, not to diet rashly and incur rapid weight loss which can be as destructive biologically as being overweight. This always leads to weight gain when you've stopped dieting.

- Feeling happier, healthier and fitter than ever before and also setting a good example and feeding my son a healthier diet.

- Since losing all my weight, my confidence has been boosted (slightly). I feel fitter and healthier. Exercise seems easier for me now I'm lighter. The fear of going back to how I was motivates me to eat healthily.

- If I put on an item of clothing that I previously felt good in and now I feel it's a bit tight – the alarm bells ring, cut out the chips!

- If see a photo of myself and I look overweight... it drags down your self-confidence

- My work means I am in front of new people presenting/selling/managing on a daily basis, therefore self-confidence is vital to my success. My self-confidence partly comes from being comfortable in my skin and with my self-image, I can then just focus on what the brain should be doing!

- If I eat lots of 'rubbish' food I feel sluggish and disappointed in myself – I don't like that feeling!

Introduction

- *I love exercise so I find it easy to be active.*

- *I want to be an active mum so I can play and enjoy life with my son for as long as possible, and I want to teach him good, healthy lifestyle habits so he can do the same for his children in time.*

- *I want to feel confident in my clothes and on holiday.*

- *I know if I go for a run or do some exercise I ALWAYS feel better/happier for it.*

- *I like to look and feel healthy, much of my self-esteem comes from feeling fit, healthy and looking in shape so that motivates me to make the effort.*

What advice would you give to someone who is overweight and why?

- *Be sensible – if you want to lose weight, do it gradually and don't be overambitious. Combine your diet with exercise – but again, take it gradually.*

- *Don't buy treats and junk food so it is not in the house to tempt you. Have something (healthy) to drink when you feel hungry as it sometimes could be dehydration not hunger you are feeling. Find a physical activity you really enjoy and doing that may curb the craving to overeat/eat junk food and make you feel better about yourself.*

- *Working out the calories that go into your body compared to the calories you burn daily was the only thing that worked for me. The first two weeks were really hard and the results were not instant. But get past the first two weeks and it gets easier. Just persevere and you will see the results.*

- *Cut out the rubbish! i.e. chocolate and crisps – just don't buy that sort of food for home, if the temptation isn't there then you can't indulge.*

- *Fill your time and get busy – don't give yourself the spare time to think about food*

- DON'T tell yourself you're on a diet. If ever I do this, my time is spent working out what I can eat next... just consciously select healthier options.

- Be active in life even if you can't get to the gym...walk to the shop instead of drive, park in the furthest spot away in the car park rather than parking up right outside the door.

- In my office I purposely don't have a printer on my desk, it's in the office next door so I have to get up and move around every so often to go and get my printing! Crazy but otherwise it would be easy to sit at my desk for 10 hours solid – every step counts!

- Exercise makes me feel happy, increases my self-esteem and confidence so even if I'm feeling not my 'ideal weight' I think a positive attitude and mindset can make a person very attractive to others and to themselves.

- If you set yourself a goal stick with it and don't cheat but don't be overambitious in setting a goal; it's got to be achievable.

- Use a friend, neighbour, buddy to help you and encourage you. Talk about it. You're trying to better yourself and no one will be negative about that so share your thoughts and feelings and people/friends/family will support you.

- Get a dog, since having mine I walk twice a day every day so I know I am at least reasonably fit.

- Set some realistic goals for healthy eating, weight loss and exercise. Keep reminding yourself of the reasons and benefits and that the effort will be worth it. Make sure you have the right people supporting, motivating and helping you.

Part 1

Weight Loss

Introduction

In the developed world more and more people are becoming overweight and obese and this trend is set to continue. There are numerous health problems associated with being overweight that can include physical, mental and emotional health conditions, yet in virtually all cases these issues are self-inflicted. We are responsible for our weight as a result of the choices we make, particularly in respect of what we eat and drink and how physically active we are.

As a general rule our weight is determined by what we eat and drink, through the consumption of calories and how much physical activity we do in terms of burning off those calories. If our calories in are greater than our calories out then inevitably we will put on weight. And as we will see being overweight can lead to many health issues.

This section looks to explore most of the issues that can be caused by being overweight, providing greater knowledge and understanding of the risks and consequences, which will hopefully make people more aware and motivate them to make healthier choices and lead a healthier and happier life.

Being overweight – the issues

There are a range of issues that may be caused as a result of being overweight, and the more overweight you are the greater the risks. Everyone is aware that being overweight and obese is 'unhealthy' but many people won't know about all the potential dangers that can affect your physical, mental and emotional health and how this can impact on all aspects of your life.

Once you understand, are aware and have the knowledge regarding the issues of being overweight you are much more likely to be able to do something positive about it and be motivated to make changes that will be beneficial to you and people close to you. So please read through carefully and be honest with yourself. I am sure you want to be healthier and happier and that can definitely happen.

Physical health

Overweight and obesity may increase the risk of many health problems, including diabetes, heart disease and certain cancers. Also, if you are pregnant, excess weight may lead to short- and long-term health problems for you and your child.

This section tells you more about the links between excess weight and many health conditions. It also explains how reaching and maintaining a normal weight may help you and people you care about stay healthier as you get older.

How can I tell if I weigh too much?

Knowing two numbers may help you understand your risk: your body mass index (BMI) score and your waist size in inches.

The BMI is one way to tell whether you are at a normal weight, are overweight, or are obese. It measures your weight in relation to your height and provides a score to help place you in a category:

Part 1 – Weight Loss

- normal weight: BMI of 18.5 to 24.9
- overweight: BMI of 25 to 29.9
- obesity: BMI of 30 or higher

$$BMI = weight\ (kg) \div by\ height\ (m)^2$$

Example 1: 85kg and 1.80 metres

$85 \div 3.24 =$ **26.23** (in the overweight category)

Example 2: 90kg and 1.70 metres

$90 \div 2.89 =$ **31.14** (in the obesity category)

Another important number to know is your waist size in inches. Having too much fat around your waist may increase health risks even more than having fat in other parts of your body.

Women with a waist size of more than 35 inches and men with a waist size of more than 40 inches may have higher chances of developing diseases related to obesity.

Type 2 diabetes

Type 2 diabetes is a disease in which blood-sugar levels are above normal. High blood sugar is a major cause of heart disease, kidney disease, stroke, amputation and blindness. In 2009, diabetes was the seventh leading cause of death in the United States.

Type 2 diabetes is the most common type of diabetes. Family history and genes play a large role in the condition, and other risk factors include a low activity level, poor diet and excess body weight around the waist.

About 80 percent of people with type 2 diabetes are overweight or obese. It isn't clear why people who are overweight are more likely to develop this disease. It may be that being overweight causes cells to change, making them resistant to the hormone insulin. Insulin carries sugar from the blood to the cells, where it is used for energy. When a person is insulin-resistant, blood sugar cannot be taken up by the cells, resulting in high blood sugar. In addition, the cells that produce insulin must work extra hard to try to keep blood sugar normal. This may cause these cells gradually to fail.

If you are at risk for type 2 diabetes, losing weight may help prevent or delay the onset of the condition. If you have type 2 diabetes, losing weight and becoming more physically active can help you control your blood-sugar levels and prevent or delay health problems. Losing weight and exercising more may also allow you to reduce the amount of diabetes medicine you take.

High blood pressure

Every time your heart beats, it pumps blood through your arteries to the rest of your body. Blood pressure is how hard your blood pushes against the walls of your arteries. High blood pressure (hypertension) usually has no symptoms, but it may cause serious problems, such as heart disease, stroke and kidney failure.

A blood pressure of 120/80 mm Hg (often referred to as '120 over 80') is considered normal. If the top number (systolic blood pressure) is consistently 140 or higher, or the bottom number (diastolic blood pressure) is 90 or higher, you are considered to have high blood pressure.

High blood pressure is linked to overweight and obesity in several ways. Having a large body size may increase blood pressure because your heart needs to pump harder to supply blood to all your cells. Excess fat may also damage your kidneys, which help regulate blood pressure.

Weight loss that will get you close to the normal BMI range may greatly lower high blood pressure. Other helpful changes are to quit smoking, reduce salt and get regular physical activity. However, if lifestyle changes aren't enough, your doctor may prescribe drugs to lower your blood pressure.

Heart disease

Heart disease is a term used to describe several problems that may affect your heart. The most common problem happens when a blood vessel that carries blood to the heart becomes hard and narrow. This may prevent the heart from getting all the blood it needs. Other problems may affect how well the heart pumps. If you have heart disease, you may suffer from a heart attack, heart failure, sudden cardiac death, angina (chest pain) or abnormal heart rhythm. Heart disease is the leading cause of death in Britain and the United States.

People who are overweight or obese often have health problems that may increase the risk for heart disease. These health problems include high blood pressure, high cholesterol and high blood sugar. In addition, excess weight may cause changes to your heart that make it work harder to send blood to all the cells in your body.

Losing 5 to 10 percent of your weight may lower your chances of developing heart disease. If you weigh 200 pounds, this means losing as little as 10 pounds. Weight loss may improve blood pressure, cholesterol levels and blood flow.

Stroke

A stroke happens when the flow of blood to a part of your brain stops, causing brain cells to die. The most common type of stroke, called ischemic stroke, occurs when a blood clot blocks an artery that carries blood to the brain. Another type of stroke, called haemorrhagic stroke, happens when a blood vessel in the brain bursts.

Overweight and obesity are known to increase blood pressure. High blood pressure is the leading cause of strokes. Excess weight also increases your chances of developing other problems linked to strokes, including high cholesterol, high blood sugar and heart disease.

One of the most important things you can do to reduce your stroke risk is to keep your blood pressure under control. Losing weight may help you lower your blood pressure. It may also improve your cholesterol and blood-sugar levels, which may then lower your risk for stroke.

Cancer

Being overweight increases the risk of developing certain cancers, including:

Breast, colon, rectum, endometrium (lining of uterus), gall bladder and kidney

Cancer occurs when cells in one part of the body, such as the colon, grow abnormally or out of control and these cancerous cells will sometimes spread to other parts of the body, such as the liver. Cancer is the second leading cause of death in the United States.

Gaining weight as an adult increases the risk for several cancers, even if the weight gain doesn't result in overweight or obesity. It isn't known exactly how being overweight increases cancer risk. Fat cells may release hormones that affect cell growth, leading to cancer. Also, eating or physical activity habits that may lead to being overweight may also contribute to cancer risk.

Avoiding weight gain may prevent a rise in cancer risk. Healthy eating and good physical activity habits may lower cancer risk, and weight loss may also lower your risk.

Sleep apnoea

Sleep apnoea is a condition in which a person has one or more pauses in breathing during sleep. A person who has sleep apnoea may suffer from daytime sleepiness, difficulty focusing and even heart failure.

Obesity is the most important risk factor for sleep apnoea. A person who is overweight may have more fat stored around his or her neck. This may make the airway smaller, which can make breathing difficult or loud (because of snoring), or breathing may stop altogether for short periods of time. In addition, fat stored in the neck and throughout the body may produce substances that cause inflammation. Inflammation in the neck is a risk factor for sleep apnoea.

Weight loss usually improves sleep apnoea. Weight loss may help to decrease neck size and lessen inflammation. Other sleep issues can also be caused by being overweight and obese, and poor sleep can lead to many other health problems.

Osteoarthritis

Osteoarthritis is a common health problem that causes pain and stiffness in the joints. It is often related to ageing or to an injury, and most often affects the joints of the hands, knees, hips and lower back.

Being overweight is one of the risk factors for osteoarthritis, along with joint injury, older age and genetic factors. Extra weight may place extra pressure on joints and cartilage (the hard but slippery tissue that covers the ends of your bones at a joint), causing them to wear away. In addition, people with more body fat may have higher levels of substances in the blood that cause inflammation, and inflamed joints may raise the risk for osteoarthritis.

For those who are overweight or obese, losing weight may help reduce the risk of developing osteoarthritis. Loss of at least 5 percent of your body weight may decrease stress on your knees, hips and lower back, and lessen inflammation in your body.

If you have osteoarthritis, losing weight may help improve your symptoms. Research also shows that exercise is one of the best treatments for osteoarthritis; it can improve mood, decrease pain and increase flexibility.

Liver disease

Fatty liver disease, also known as non-alcoholic steatohepatitis (NASH), occurs when fat builds up in the liver and causes injury. Fatty liver disease may lead to severe liver damage, cirrhosis (scar tissue) or even liver failure.

Fatty liver disease usually produces mild or no symptoms. It is like alcoholic liver disease, but it isn't caused by alcohol and can occur in people who drink little or no alcohol.

The cause of fatty liver disease is still not really understood. It most often affects people who are middle-aged, overweight or obese, and/or diabetic, although fatty liver disease may also affect children.

Although there is no specific treatment for fatty liver disease, patients are generally advised to lose weight, eat a healthy diet, increase physical activity and avoid drinking alcohol. If you have fatty liver disease, lowering your body weight to a healthy range may improve liver tests and reverse the disease to some extent.

Kidney disease

Your kidneys are two bean-shaped organs that filter blood, removing extra water and waste products, which become urine. Your kidneys also help control blood pressure so that your body can stay healthy.

Kidney disease means that the kidneys are damaged and can't filter blood like they should. This damage can cause wastes to build up in the body. It can also cause other problems that can harm your health.

Obesity increases the risk of diabetes and high blood pressure, the most common causes of chronic kidney disease. Recent studies suggest that even in the absence of these risks, obesity itself may promote chronic kidney disease and quicken its progress.

If you are in the early stages of chronic kidney disease, losing weight may slow the disease and keep your kidneys healthier longer. You should also choose foods with less salt (sodium), keep your blood pressure under control and keep your blood glucose in the target range.

Pregnancy problems

Overweight and obesity raise the risk of health problems for both mother and baby that may occur during pregnancy. Pregnant women who are overweight or obese may have an increased risk for

- developing gestational diabetes (high blood sugar during pregnancy)
- having pre-eclampsia (high blood pressure during pregnancy that can cause severe problems for both mother and baby if left untreated)
- needing a C-section and, as a result, taking longer to recover after giving birth

Babies of overweight or obese mothers are at an increased risk of being born too soon, being stillborn (dead in the womb after 20 weeks of pregnancy), and having neural tube defects (defects of the brain and spinal cord).

Pregnant women who are overweight are more likely to develop insulin resistance, high blood sugar and high blood pressure. Being overweight also increases the risks associated with surgery and anaesthesia, and severe obesity increases surgery time and blood loss.

Gaining too much weight during pregnancy can have long-term effects for both mother and child. These effects include the mother having overweight or obesity after the child is born. Another risk is that the baby may gain too much weight later as a child or as an adult.

If you are pregnant talk to your doctor or health care provider about how much weight gain is right for you during pregnancy and if you are overweight or obese and would like to become pregnant, talk to your doctor about losing weight first and about being active during pregnancy. Reaching a normal weight before becoming pregnant may reduce your chances of developing weight-related problems.

Losing excess weight after delivery may help women reduce their health risks. For example, if a woman develops gestational diabetes, losing weight may lower her risk of developing diabetes later in life.

How can I lower my risk of health problems related to being overweight?

If you are considered to be overweight, losing as little as 5 percent of your body weight may lower your risk for several diseases, including heart disease and type 2 diabetes. If you weigh 200 pounds, this means losing 10 pounds. Slow and steady weight loss of ½ to 2 pounds per week, and not more than 3 pounds per week, is the safest way to lose weight.

Guidelines on physical activity recommend that you get at least 150 minutes a week of moderate aerobic activity (like biking or brisk walking). To lose weight, or to maintain weight loss, you may need to be active for up to 300 minutes per week. You also need to do activities to strengthen muscles (like push-ups or sit-ups) at least twice a week.

Read through the 'How to lose weight' and 'Healthy eating' sections to gain greater knowledge and understanding so you will be better placed to lose weight if that is needed. Also, look to increase your physical activity and exercise levels.

You will find another helpful book available in this series called *The Real Benefits of Exercise*.

Emotional health

The above section outlined many areas of physical health that can be at risk due to being overweight, but there are also many emotional health issues that can affect people, often on a daily basis. There is the saying 'you are what you eat', but also it is often true to say that 'you feel what you eat', as being overweight can affect you in a variety of other ways that impact on your life and happiness.

Confidence and self-esteem

For many people who are overweight their confidence and self-esteem can be affected in a negative way. Lower confidence and lower self-esteem result directly from being overweight and also indirectly from a range of factors that being overweight can affect. Confidence and self-esteem play a huge role in how happy we are in our lives and can be both the cause and effect of a number of issues. The more confident we are the more likely we are to try new things, go to new places, meet new people, achieve and accomplish more, believe we can succeed in something and generally live a more fulfilling, successful and satisfying life. If we don't achieve what we want, if we don't look how we would like to, if we get criticised and judged negatively by others and are not who we want to be, then our confidence decreases. The same can apply to self-esteem.

If we are overweight and do not want to be then there is a good chance that it will lower our confidence and self-esteem in these ways and will continue to have an effect as long as we are in that position. You may be very happy and content with many other aspects of your life, but those will also be affected as a consequence, so the effect of being overweight is compounded far more than the actual issue itself. On the positive side, if you are overweight and do things that help reduce your weight, and you see and feel the difference, then your confidence and self-esteem are likely to increase quite quickly, hopefully motivating you to continue with the weight loss

Another book in this series focuses on confidence and may be helpful to read. It is called *Understanding & Building Confidence*.

Depression

For some people becoming depressed can lead to putting on additional weight and for some people being overweight can be a factor contributing to depression. Either way there can be a relationship between the two, and neither is good for us or are desirable conditions. If being overweight is one of the effects of depression then this will potentially lead to many issues caused by being overweight. If depression is an effect of being overweight then the depression will become the cause of many other issues.

Although being overweight is unlikely to be the main cause or underlying reason for someone becoming depressed, it can certainly make things worse and will make it harder to prevent, manage or overcome depression. Many unhealthy foods can play a role in causing depression, lack of exercise and activity can be a factor, low self-esteem and low confidence associated with being overweight will not help and there can be many other knock-on effects that can all contribute to depressive feelings and behaviours, which can become a vicious negative circle, making it harder to stop.

There is another book in this series that looks at many aspects of how to prevent and manage depression, called *Managing Stress & Preventing Depression*.

Anxiety

Many people suffer with varying degrees of anxiety which can cause many issues and potentially can also impact on their weight. However, being overweight can actually contribute to feeling anxious, prolong the condition and make the anxiety worse. A lot of people who are overweight do not feel comfortable about their size and appearance and worry about what other people think of them. Most forms and levels of anxiety are concerned with what other people think about the person affected, so if this is the case then being overweight will add to the anxiety and may be a significant factor in how they think.

People with anxiety are more likely to jump to conclusions in a negative way, be more paranoid, overthink situations and comments, take things out of context and be overly worried about how others perceive them. Not being comfortable with how you look or not feeling very fit, sporty or active is only likely to add to any underlying anxiety issues.

Isolation

For some people who are overweight and uncomfortable with how they look a further issue may arise, potentially alongside increased anxiety, and that is they become more isolated, withdrawn and reclusive, not wanting to go out and socialise, or meet up with friends, family or colleagues, and keeping themselves hidden away.

By becoming more isolated it is likely this will only reduce confidence and self-esteem further, which in turn is more likely to cause someone to 'comfort eat' and be less active and thus put on more weight. It can become a downward spiral whereby the situation gets worse, the weight increases and the negative consequences escalate. Humans are generally very social creatures and it is healthy to mix, communicate and meet up with other people, so if this does not happen you are likely to become unhealthier and also find it harder to regain the confidence to be social again.

Stigma

Although the numbers of people being overweight and obese are rising and it is more common to see 'larger' people, there can still be a stigma associated with it and this can cause further issues. Someone who is overweight may get called names, be sneered at, looked at in a disapproving way and may be overlooked for certain opportunities or left out of activities.

Regarding work and employment, someone's weight may be a factor at a job interview, a potential promotion, a social event or at a team meeting. There could also be bullying or discrimination because of someone's size and appearance. Although this shouldn't happen or be allowed to happen they are real possibilities that cannot be ignored.

Additionally, a person's size or physical capability may prevent them from doing various things and therefore lead to them missing out on opportunities both at work and in their personal life. People can gain confidence and improve self-esteem by achieving things, having a purpose, being fulfilled and taking part in beneficial activities. If your weight prevents this or limits the opportunities then it can become a problem and you will miss out on many things that could make you happier as well as healthier. It can then become a vicious negative circle that is hard to get out of and unhealthy habits, both physical and emotional, can develop, further compounding those issues.

Setting an example for our children

One of the biggest concerns in our modern society is the rise of health issues including obesity levels in children. Each year the percentage of children who are overweight or obese continues to increase, and as we have seen, with that come many potential issues for their physical, mental and emotional health.

There are a wide range of reasons for this worrying trend but it cannot help if children see adults and in particular their own parents being overweight as a result of eating a poor diet and not being very active. It is much more difficult to encourage our children to eat healthily and be active or to insist on them maintaining a healthy weight if they see their parents, teachers, family members, mentors, etc., being overweight themselves.

Setting a good example to our children in all aspects of life will make a positive difference to their lives as they will learn better habits and become healthier as a result. Rather than just talking the talk with them about food and exercise and being healthy, if you are also able to walk the walk it will make a big difference that will be beneficial for you as well as the children, so hopefully we can reverse the worrying trend and instead see the next generation being better informed, having an improved understanding about weight issues and forming positive habits so they become healthier and happier.

It's not all about your weight and weight loss!

This section of the book has focused on weight loss and the issues around being overweight and obese as that is generally where there are many more problems relating to health, and it is a growing and worsening issue. However, it isn't always about your weight and there are many healthy people who would be classed as overweight and many unhealthy people who are underweight or indeed at what would be called a good weight. When it comes to health – physical, mental and emotional – there are a wide range of relevant factors and your weight, although important, is usually just one of these. So make sure you consider your overall health and wellbeing and how your weight may affect this.

You can be 'overweight' and healthy

Some people who would be classed as overweight and have a high BMI score are actually very healthy, so be careful not to base assessments of health on just weight. For example, nearly all professional rugby players would be deemed 'overweight' if they took the conventional BMI tests, yet they would score very highly on most aspects of their health. Muscle does weigh more than fat, so the actual make-up of your body tissues and the percentage of muscle versus fat is a factor.

Also, you may be someone who is overweight but you don't smoke or drink alcohol and you do some level of exercise. In this case it is likely that you are generally 'healthier' than someone of a good weight who smokes, drinks alcohol and does very little physical activity. There are many measures of health, many aspects of health and many contributing factors, so be careful not to focus everything on your weight if you want to be healthier and happier.

Risks of being 'underweight'

There are also health dangers with being underweight and this must not be ignored. Although the levels are much lower, there are still significant numbers of people who have 'underweight' issues, usually caused by not eating enough and not eating the right types of food. Often there is pressure from the media, peer groups and society in general to look a certain way and this can also be very damaging to your physical, mental and emotional health if as a result you become underweight.

Many eating disorders exist for both men and woman that can lead to being underweight, for example bulimia and anorexia. If your body is not getting the nutrients, minerals, proteins, fats, glucose and other ingredients it needs then this will damage your health. If you have issues in this respect then please consult your doctor and seek advice, and try to understand the causes and also the risks to your health of being underweight.

How to put on weight

Some people may be underweight and wish to put weight on and there are health risks in doing this. Similarly to losing weight the advice is to be as knowledgeable as possible, take a sensible, steady approach and do not try to gain weight too quickly. Rapid weight gain can be very unhealthy, especially as your body will not be used to the high calorie intake and it is likely that many of the foods will be high in sugar, fat and salt.

As muscle weighs more than fat and is generally much healthier, then it would be advised that in order to gain weight more protein needs to be consumed, because this is the main fuel needed to grow and rebuild muscle tissue. Using free weights or gym equipment can be effective in building muscle mass combined with additional protein and calorie intake. However, if you feel the need to put on weight it is advisable to consult with your doctor, do more research and potentially discuss it with both a nutritionist and fitness advisor.

Why are so many people overweight?

It's important to try and understand why so many people are overweight and why this is increasing in our society. There are of course many factors and some are more relevant than others but to tackle the issue, both individuals and society have to explore all the possible factors and see how best to address them in order to make a positive difference. The many factors include the following:

We eat too much

A very obvious reason why people are overweight is that they eat too much. There are many reasons as to why people eat too much, which really need to be looked at and understood.

In a very primitive way humans are wired to eat when they can and effectively store food in case of emergencies – mainly being whether we need energy available for certain physical activities or we may not have food available to us for some time. For hundreds of thousands of years this was very necessary for survival as humans developed and evolved. Our distant ancestors wouldn't always have food sources available to them and could go days without eating much, so needed the reserves. Additionally they may have come under threat by animals or other humans and needed to have reserves of energy to run or fight for their survival or to go out and hunt animals for more food.

So in this respect it makes a lot of sense that when food became available humans would look to take advantage and indulge themselves in as much food as possible, basically for their own survival. And this behaviour is pretty hard-wired into our brains and physiology since we don't evolve as quickly as the developments we make as a human race in many forms.

In the modern, developed world it is very unlikely that we would not have access to food all the time if needed. How often have you been in a position in which you really didn't know where your next meal might come from, or not have any access to food? Our lives are completely different now and we generally have 24-hour access to food sources, so we are never in a position where we could go one, two or more days without food. Additionally, we are no longer put in positions of danger where we need energy reserves in order to run away or fight for our survival. Energy reserves nowadays are really for optional physical activities we may choose to participate in.

So when we eat now we don't need to indulge and eat more than necessary to build up reserves, yet our brain is still telling us to eat more just in case! It is important to understand this and to try to manage the brain's instinctive nature. We have access to food at any time so we do not need to overeat and we should really be looking to eat just what is necessary for our modern lives, not our distant past 'survival' lives.

Now you could use this 'brain wired' reason for overeating as an excuse and think that this means it is not your fault and you can't help it if your brain tells you to eat more than is needed. Well yes, you could go with that mentality but it will not benefit you! It is important to be in control of your food intake and you can manage your eating behaviours in this respect.

We eat the wrong food types

Another big reason why people are overweight is because of the type of foods they eat. In a similar way to the general notion that the brain is wired to eat more than it needs to, as explained in the previous section, our brain also craves more of the food types that are best for energy and energy reserve storage. These food types are more of the carbohydrates that generally contain the most calories and provide the most energy. So on the basis that we need energy and energy reserves to survive, our brain often targets and craves these far more than other food types.

Food types such as breads, cakes, sweets, chocolate, crisps, cereals, etc., are more likely to have that 'pull' effect on us as they provide the most calories and energy. However, we very rarely need this energy either in the present or as storage for the future so inevitably if we eat these foods we put on weight. So eating the wrong type of food can have a big effect on our weight as we don't need to eat these food types, and combined with eating too much it is no real surprise that so many people are overweight nowadays.

If we are using the energy and burning the calories straight away, perhaps from doing an exhausting physical challenge, then those food types can be very beneficial as they provide an instant energy source and will be burnt off and not stored by the body. So it is wrong to say that these food types are necessarily bad or wrong for us, just that more often than not we do not burn the calories off. Additionally, they only really provide one key benefit, which is energy, and have very little other nutritional value or benefit to our health.

So the basic rule is that if you are requiring energy in the very short term and will burn off the calories then carbohydrates are fine and can be very beneficial for those activities. However, if you will not be burning off the calories and using the energy then you will almost certainly put on weight and be eating far more than you need, and thus the body will store this ultimately as fat.

A further big effect of these carbohydrates, particularly ones high in sugar content, is that unless you are burning off the calories and being active at the time, you will probably feel more tired after the initial boost and thus more likely to look for an 'energy boosting' pick-me-up, which is likely to be more food and more sugar and carbohydrates! It can become a vicious circle whereby you eat then feel tired then eat again then feel tired and eat again and so on. Your blood-sugar levels tend to increase rapidly on consumption and you feel that 'fix' , 'high' or energy spike and then fairly quickly your blood-sugar levels drop, which can make you feel lethargic and in need of more energy.

If you are able to keep your blood-sugar levels more constant and eat less sugar and fewer carbohydrates then you will generally feel less tired and not have the urge for more food and an energy boost.

'The key to healthy eating? Avoid any food that has a TV commercial!'

Sugar addiction

Over the last few decades there has been a huge increase in sugar consumption, which has led to both an increase in overweight and many people becoming sugar addicts. There are two main reasons why there has been such a massive increase in sugar in our foods and drinks – firstly sugar is very cheap, and secondly it can be very addictive. Food and drink manufacturers benefit enormously from these two reasons and therefore sugar is prevalent in so much of what we eat and drink. To increase sales and profits it is therefore in manufacturers' interests to use sugar in vast quantities and in so many products. Very few will care about our health and there is no incentive to reduce or stop with the huge sugar content.

Governments have seemingly only recently realised the significant health issues and costs to public health as a result of sugar, yet there is little they can do or will do. Unless serious action is taken to educate people and manufacturers, together with tougher regulations then the problem will only continue and worsen.

Because sugar is a cheap ingredient for manufacturers and it is addictive, so many of the special offers, bargains, deals, fun adverts, colourful attractive packaging, etc., are on these products. People love a bargain, are enticed by the advertising and promotions and of course many people love the taste and the feeling, as well as many being addicted.

In some ways sugar should be seen as a drug because of its addictive qualities and the effect it has. Many people have strong cravings for a sugar 'hit' and need their 'fix', and once they have had the sugar they get a short-term 'high' that makes them feel good. However, like most drugs this soon wears off and can leave people feeling worse, lacking energy and lower in mood. They have a blood-sugar high followed by a blood-sugar low.

Sugar is often associated with giving us energy and indeed sugar in its various formats can provide us quickly and effectively with the glucose energy our body and organs, including the brain, need. However, if that glucose energy is not used then the body will store it and put it into our 'reserves' for later use. Most people will not use the energy at the time or in the future and these 'reserves' build up by converting to fats stored in our body and around our internal organs. Of course, over time this builds and builds if our sugar intake continues.

Another factor is that in many of the 'low-fat' products seen in our shops and on our shelves today, there is a huge amount of sugar. Manufacturers can fool people with apparently healthy 'low-fat' products, yet they contain large amounts of sugar which inevitably turns into fat in our body. So be very careful and aware and look closely at the food labelling and ingredients on both foods and drinks. The recommended daily amount of sugar is no more than 60g and that works out at 15 teaspoons per day. So try to calculate your sugar intake from foods and drinks and remember that unless you are using that energy it will end up in your body being stored as fat.

Lack of exercise and activity

Another main reason for people being overweight is a lack of exercise and physical activity. At a very basic level we require food for energy so that our bodies, organs and brain can function. For most of the time humans have been on the planet they have had to be very physically active, primarily to find food in order to survive; walking and running many miles per day to find water, as well as fruit, nuts, vegetables, etc., and also to hunt animals. The simple equation was that if you weren't active and moving then you wouldn't find food and would not survive.

In our modern life it is perfectly possible to survive if necessary without leaving the front door of your house! We no longer have to walk for miles in search of food or run for hours hunting down animals. We don't even have to walk to the shops to get our food any more. So our 'need' to exercise is no longer there and when given the choice most people do not exercise, and limit their physical activity to a minimum.

If we are not active as much then we require fewer calories and therefore less food to survive, yet if we eat as much as we used to need or in fact more than we used to need, then the obvious outcome is that we put on weight because we are not burning those additional calories and using them for fuel.

There are many other issues and problems that result from a lack of exercise and activity, but focusing on the weight issue it is a clear and growing problem that people are becoming more overweight as they do less and less exercise and physical activity.

Furthermore, exercise can increase your metabolism, which increases the rate of calorie burning beyond the actual activity time, so with a higher metabolism you are likely to be less overweight than if you have a low metabolism. So exercise and activity shouldn't be looked at for just the benefits at the time but for an overall, longer range of benefit in terms of the weight-loss equation that will be looked at later in the book.

'Let exercise be your stress reliever, not food.'

Stress, depression and anxiety

Many people are being affected by stress, depression and anxiety and these numbers are continuing to rise in the modern, western world with approximately one in five people in the UK directly affected. Although they can be looked at and seen rightly as three separate conditions there is often a strong overlap and correlation between them and a lot of people will suffer with all three conditions. There are many contributing factors that cause the conditions, and many effects and symptoms related to all three.

A poor diet, comfort eating, lack of exercise, poor sleep and drinking excessively can all lead to weight gain. Many of these habits can form as a result of stress, depression and anxiety issues. Lacking motivation, feeling tired, a lowering of confidence, poor self-worth, feeling overwhelmed, unable to find the time, not feeling social, becoming withdrawn and reclusive and generally not feeling good about yourself or your situation will all add to the problems and can cause weight issues.

If any or all of these three conditions affect you and play a part in you being overweight then it is important to try and tackle the causes and underlying problems of these. In turn, your weight issues are likely to improve. It is important you work out the causes and effects and focus on dealing more with the causes. There is a lot of help available in many areas and if some of these underlying reasons are addressed and worked on effectively then many people will as a result have fewer problems with their weight.

I would recommend reading the book *Managing Stress & Preventing Depression*, which is available as part of this series.

Habit, choices and excuses

Humans are often referred to as creatures of habit and very often this is true, as we are very good at making things habitual, whether that's good or bad. Unfortunately, in recent decades our habits when it comes to food and eating have become worse and are seemingly continuing to worsen. Those harmful habits need to be addressed and changed into more beneficial and positive eating habits.

These bad habits include not cooking but instead buying 'microwave' food, ready meals, processed food, take-away meals, and eating out, snacking on crisps and chocolate, etc. There are so many bad habits that may at first creep in but then become more frequent and can eventually become more the norm than the exception.

Habits are effectively formed by the choices we make and we all have choices when it comes to the food and drink we consume these days. We are very fortunate that there is such a wide choice of foods available and so many shops or places where we can buy the food. Yet very often, despite the very wide choices available, we choose the foods that are not healthy and also choose more food than we need. When we purchase food and when we consume food we have choices at each stage, so people should recognise that there are choices to be made and they have the opportunity to make better or worse choices. Yet often people don't recognise this and therefore don't take responsibility, which can then lead to them becoming overweight.

In addition to forming bad habits and making poor choices, many people will find excuses for being overweight and eating unhealthily; excuses such as they don't have time to eat properly or it is too expensive to eat a healthy diet or they don't know what foods are good or bad for them. Or they use excuses for lack of exercise and physical activity such as they don't have time, or it costs too much or they have an injury.

Sometimes there seem to be genuine reasons and factors but too often they are excuses, and if the person is really honest with themselves about the situation they will realise that indeed they are excuses and not genuine reasons. It is then about trying to make the better choices for themselves rather than using excuses. Making excuses can become a habit so be careful, and seek to make the good choices a habit instead.

Lack of accountability and personal responsibility

Unfortunately there are too many people who do not take accountability or personal responsibility for their own health. There are a small minority of people who have physical or mental health issues and disabilities that mean they are unable to take accountability for themselves, but the vast majority of people can and should take personal responsibility for their health. Too often society and individuals look for a cure or treatment rather than tackling the causes and trying to prevent the issues in the first place.

Millions of pounds are spent on trying to develop some kind of wonder diet pill rather than looking at the reasons why people are overweight and how it can be prevented in the first place.

In the UK, we are very fortunate to have very good health care, with the NHS accessible and available for everyone. This is not so in most countries. So although we are very privileged and lucky to have such health care and free access, it does lead to people potentially taking less personal accountability and responsibility for their health. If the NHS will fix, cure, treat, sort out and mend health issues, illnesses and disease for free then it makes sense that people value their health less. If they had to pay for the same services directly or did not have access to such great health care would they take more care of their personal health?

So many of our health issues, illnesses and diseases are self-inflicted as a result of lifestyle choices including smoking, alcohol consumption, drugs, lack of exercise and the food we consume. Many people don't understand or appreciate this, and how so many health issues can be prevented, which would mean huge financial savings for the NHS and also a huge number of illness and health problems that could be avoided. If more people were aware, had the knowledge and were able to tackle some of the factors then so many of us would be healthier and happier, and the country would save billions!

You can be healthier and happier and be a great influence for others if you take more personal responsibility for your health by becoming more knowledgeable and making more effort. You will feel healthier, more confident, be happier and do much more with your life. The rewards are worth the effort.

'Be the change you want to see in the world.' – Mahatma Gandhi

Diets – fads and fiction

Each year millions of people will attempt a 'diet' with the aim of losing weight and more often than not this is not successful, especially in the longer term. Why do diets not work? And if they do work for the short term, why do so many people then end up putting the weight back on over a longer period? There are three main reasons why, typically, diets do not work. Firstly, in terms of nutritional value and health balance the diets

Weight Loss & Healthy Eating

are often not very good for sustained weight loss. Secondly, the underlying reasons for being overweight and poor eating habits are not addressed and thirdly, the motivation to stick to a disciplined diet does not continue for long.

Crash dieting, in which you hugely cut down how much you eat, is popular because it's seen as a quick fix, but sadly there's no such thing. Crash diets might help you to lose a few pounds at first, but they won't help you to stay a healthy weight in the long run. Usually as soon as you stop restricting your calorie intake, you will put the weight straight back on again.

This happens because if you lose weight too quickly, you tend to lose a lot of lean body tissue – muscle – as well as fat. When this happens, your body starts to work more slowly, meaning that it needs fewer calories to function day to day. That's why the weight piles back on so quickly once you go back to your usual eating habits; your body has adjusted to a lower calorie intake, so the extra calories are stored as fat. If you're overweight and want to lose some, the trick is to set realistic goals. Aim to lose weight at a rate of about 0.5kg (1lb) per week.

I'm not a fan of fad diets like the 'cabbage soup diet', the 'maple syrup diet', the 'blood group diet' – no sooner does one fad diet lose popularity than another one comes along, promising to help you lose weight through one method or another. A healthy, balanced diet is essential for good health and cutting out entire food groups, as stipulated in some diets, can be dangerous. No single food contains all the nutrients and fibre you need to stay healthy, so it's important to eat a range of foods from the five main food groups.

If you're trying to lose weight, rather than cut something out completely, try to eat less fat and sugar and replace them with more of other food groups, such as fruit and vegetables. Weight for weight, fat has more than twice the calories of carbohydrates and protein. Try to find low-fat alternatives to creamy sauces and buttery toppings, and choose cooking methods that keep the overall fat content low.

Also watch out for 'reduced-fat' foods. These may not be low in fat at all – a 'reduced-fat' product must just have a third less fat than the standard product, so it may still be high in fat ('75 percent fat-free' still means the food is a quarter fat). Alternatively, the product may contain lots of salt and sugar. Although diets such as the Atkins diet advocate cutting out fruit and vegetables, it's important to aim to include at least five portions of these in your daily diet. Not only are fruit and vegetables rich in essential vitamins, minerals and fibre, but steamed, boiled or raw, they are both filling and low in calories.

Poor sleep

Poor sleep is an issue for many people and these sleep-related issues can also affect our weight and can be a factor in people being overweight and obese. If you don't get enough sleep, or the sleep you do get is of poor quality, then you are likely to experience a wide range of effects that can impact on your health. An obvious consequence is lacking energy and feeling lethargic, which can often lead to eating more than necessary, eating the wrong types of food and being less physically active, all of which can impact negatively on our weight.

If you do less exercise and are not as physically active because of poor sleep then you will burn fewer calories and your metabolism is likely to be lower. If you feel tired you are more likely to go for the 'energy' foods, which will often contain a lot of sugar and fats providing a lot of calories that you will not burn off. In addition, by eating these foods, feeling tired and doing less exercise you are more likely to feel depressed, have a lower mood, and be more stressed, agitated and generally grumpy, which in turn will make you more likely to 'comfort eat' and thus put on weight this way too.

So if you are someone who does not sleep effectively then try to tackle this issue, because improving your sleep will have a positive effect on your weight in lots of ways.

There is another book in this series that is recommended, called *How to Sleep Better!* (available from Amazon, iBooks and iTunes).

Boredom

Often, some of the things we do that are unhealthy for us are as a result of boredom. That could be smoking, drinking, watching television, playing computer games and could also include eating! Many people eat too much and too often out of boredom. There are so many reasons why people may eat too much and become overweight but overeating because of boredom really is a poor excuse.

Tackling boredom should be relatively straightforward if some time is taken to recognise this as the issue and then to put in place strategies to combat it, which should then prevent the extra, unnecessary eating. Think about what things interest you, excite you, make you smile, etc., and look to do more of those. Do you have a passion or a hobby, and if not then is there anything that could fit that role? If you have time on your hands then look to buy healthier food and then take time to cook it. Perhaps you could prepare some healthy dishes and freeze them so you have them available for other mealtimes.

Start changing your habits, do more things that interest you, value your time more and maybe use the time to do some physical activity. Recognise if you do eat out of boredom and put in place measures to avoid it; it will soon become much easier, especially if you make better use of your time, and you will eat less.

I'm not hungry, but I am bored. Therefore I shall eat!

Obesity becoming normalised in society

Unfortunately, the number of people who are overweight and obese continues to increase, with the latest figures showing that approximately two-thirds of people in the UK are overweight and approximately a quarter are considered to be obese. Every year more people will become heavier than their 'healthy' weight and the gap between the 'healthy' weight and the average weight continues to grow wider. Apart from all the issues associated with being overweight, another factor that contributes to people being overweight is that it becomes more 'normal' and is seen more commonly. This has an impact because many will see being overweight as nothing unusual, and as a consequence they will often see it as less of an issue.

There is no question that if you go out into any town centre on any day of the week you will see far more 'overweight' and 'obese' people than you would have done say twenty years ago. If more and more people are overweight then it becomes more accepted in society and effectively normalised, and there is little incentive to manage your weight and make the effort to be at a healthy weight. And as long as the rates continue to grow and more people are overweight then the likelihood is that this will only help to increase these rates further.

Part 1 – Weight Loss

Of course, there are many factors as to why people are overweight and in order to try and reduce these numbers and stop the growing trend there needs to be plenty of help. However, in a society where people naturally compare themselves to others it becomes even harder to reduce rates when so many people are visibly overweight. People are more likely to make an effort and reduce their weight if they are encouraged, motivated, incentivised and educated on the wide range of health benefits, but if they see all around them a growing trend of people being overweight and obesity rates growing then it becomes much harder.

Losing weight

We have looked at a wide range of factors as to why so many people are overweight and these should all be considered when discussing how best to lose weight if that is your goal, or if you are looking to help others lose weight. Some of these factors may not apply but many of them will and it is important to be very honest when considering each of them.

In this section we now look at the many factors that need to be thought about and applied so that you have the best opportunity to lose weight in the right way – healthily and sustainably. Read through each carefully – you may want to have a pen handy to highlight certain areas or jot down factors on a separate notepad that you think are most relevant.

Sensible approach

Generally for the best long-term results with weight loss it is important to make whatever you do form part of your lifestyle in a way that is sustainable. This means being sensible and realistic in your goals and how long they will take as well as doing things in a healthy and safe way. Too many people attempt to lose weight with unrealistic goals or timeframes or put in place tactics that are not sustainable. We are all aware of the way that many people lose weight quickly and then it all comes back on again, sometimes even more.

To avoid this unhealthy yo-yoing, it is important to be sensible and understand how you can achieve the results you want and put in place the tools and techniques to make that happen. These may include support from others, finding what will motivate you, being more knowledgeable about your food and drink intake, having targets, finding a balance, reminding yourself of the benefits and looking at all the ways you can help yourself.

The main factors will be what you eat, how much you eat, when you eat, why you eat, how well you sleep and how much physical activity you do. These will be determined by your motivation, your knowledge and understanding, your determination, the support and encouragement you receive plus the results you see and feel. Be aware of all these and also think about the weight loss equation in a sensible and sustainable way so that it becomes easier, more natural and part of your ongoing lifestyle.

The weight-loss equation (calories)

Effectively this is the number of calories consumed less calories burned. The 'calories burned' part of the equation also needs to take into account metabolism. The higher the metabolism the more calories are burned over a longer period.

If you consumed 2,500 calories and did no exercise at all for that day and the total calories burned were 2,000, then you would have 500 calories going to your reserves thus putting on weight. Let's say you consumed 2,000 calories but did exercise that measured an additional 500 calories burned as well as the normal 2,000. This would mean you had a calorie deficit of 500 calories that would have been taken from your reserves, and thus you would be losing weight.

So if your calorie intake is less than is being burned then the body must use stored fuel for its energy. This will essentially mean your fat and muscle reserves will be being used and you will be losing weight.

Exercise will not only burn more calories directly but will generally increase your metabolism so you will continue to burn calories for longer. Steady-state metabolism rates will differ from person to person, but although a factor this is a relatively small part of the equation; far more important is the basic calories in versus calories out part. The more you are aware of, and calculate this, the more you can be in control of your weight and health.

Motivation, reasons and goals

For most people it is essential to have reasons for wanting to lose weight and be motivated to do so, otherwise it is unlikely to happen. Setting realistic, sensible and achievable goals is also going to be key to helping with the weight loss, so you need to determine what your reasons and motivations are and what goals you can set for yourself. Ask yourself what has worked before, what hasn't worked, what is most likely to work and what could potentially work.

Spend time thinking about all these different reasons and factors and seek to identify new ones that you may not have previously considered. What is really important to you?

Why do you want to lose weight? Be really honest with yourself and be realistic.

You need to be realistic because no matter who you are, you will have good and bad days. You have to have resilience but also you can't expect miracles. Once you have established good reasons and goals, write them down; keep reminding yourself of these reasons and why it is important. However hard it is and whatever the effort required, be reassured that the rewards will be worth it in terms of your overall health – physically, emotionally and mentally.

Your confidence and self-esteem will improve, you will have more energy, be able to do more things in your life, have fewer insecurities, be happier and of course, be physically healthier. It is really important that you set these goals for yourself and that your reasons are for you. Yes, other people may be a big factor in your motivation, but make sure you are doing this to improve your life first and foremost and the knock-on effect will be that other people benefit too.

There is another book in this series that may be helpful in this respect: *Motivation, Achievement & Challenges*.

The right support

Although losing weight should be about you and for you as an individual it is also really important and extremely helpful to have the right support if you can. It may not be possible and you may wish to try and do it all on your own without any outside help or support; however, if you are able to get the right support then that will undoubtedly be beneficial. At the same time, the wrong support or people will most likely have a detrimental effect so be very careful.

Think about any family, friends or colleagues who would be supportive in the right ways and help you in your goals – those people who would encourage, motivate and inspire you, and those who would want you to succeed and reach your goals, and would be supportive for weeks and months, not just a few days. Be careful of those who may not want you to succeed, may become jealous, may be a bad influence on your eating and drinking habits for example, or who have a different agenda.

Losing weight sensibly and in the right way takes time and patience as well as effort and commitment, so make sure only people who can help this way are involved and do not get wrongly influenced by those who can't.

You may find that with other people being involved you can help motivate each other, especially if each person has similar goals. You may join a group and collectively this helps, or buddy up with someone so that you can help each other. But again make sure anyone involved is the right person, and if they are not, try to get rid of them (or at least not have them involved!).

Your family may be a big factor in your progress and success, so try to ensure they are supportive, understanding and motivating. Especially with children and a partner it can be more difficult and more issues will occur on a practical level. However, if they are involved in a supportive and helpful way it will be a major factor in your success.

Be careful of the common pitfalls

There will be many reasons and factors that will determine how successful you are with your weight loss, both short and long term, plus many excuses if it doesn't work as you wanted it to. However, it is important to be aware of and understand as many potential pitfalls as possible so that you can avoid them. Different people will be affected by different pitfalls so these common areas are dealt with in no particular order. Have a careful think, though, of how likely each one is for you and your circumstances and seek to ensure that you mitigate them, avoid them or deal with them effectively.

Shops and supermarkets are generally very unhelpful, as most of the offers and bargains seem to be on unhealthy foods and drinks. Be very careful not to be influenced by these and lured in to the unhealthy special offers.

You will undoubtedly receive some bad news, have a bad day, have someone cause you grief, etc., during the weeks and months of your healthier weight-loss period. Be careful not to default to some form of comfort eating or drinking as a result. It is too easy to have the drink, the chocolate bar, the ice cream, the cake, the take-away, the chips, etc., as an answer to bad news or a bad day. Be stronger, more determined and counter the bad news by beating it with something positive, productive and healthy instead.

Peer pressure can often be a pitfall whereby actions, behaviours and views of others can have a negative effect on your goals, such as friends, family or work colleagues putting pressure on you (deliberately or not) to come out for a meal, go for drinks, have some birthday cake, cancel the gym session, etc. Be aware of this influence and pressure and work out how you can reduce it or avoid it altogether so it doesn't affect your progress.

You may well find yourself getting strong cravings for certain foods and drinks that you are trying to avoid on your weight-loss and healthy eating regime. This is quite normal and in a way you have an addiction to these, so the cravings are all part of it. How you deal with these is the key and it is best to have in place healthy alternatives or develop tools and techniques you can use in order not to 'give in' to the cravings. The longer you avoid 'the bad stuff' the easier it will become; the cravings will be much less frequent and not as strong.

Eating out, treats, celebrations and holidays

There are many temptations all around us, particularly when it comes to food, both in terms of consuming too much and in the wide range of unhealthy options available. However, despite these dangerous temptations there is also an opportunity to cut out a lot of this or reduce the downside considerably.

For many people eating out is seen as a special occasion, and also there is a sense of wanting to get value for money, so for both reasons it is far more likely that you will eat much more than you would normally, and definitely a lot more than is necessary. Perhaps you have a starter and a side roll with butter as well as your main course and maybe even a dessert too. Would you normally have that much food? Or where there is an 'all you can eat' buffet, it can often feel like a competition as to how much is it possible to consume. If you are staying at a hotel and go for breakfast, often it is the same 'all you can eat' scenario and most people take full advantage.

It is similar on holiday; both the fact that because you are on holiday it often means you can 'treat yourself' and that can mean eating a lot more unhealthy food. Plus many holidays have the 'all you can eat' buffets or the all-inclusive packages where it is literally eat and drink as much as you like. And guess what? Most people do! On average, people on an all-inclusive holiday consume approximately two and half times more calories than recommended. Of course, there is a balance to be had and yes, you are on holiday, but there really is no need to consume so much, and with some thought and a little discipline you could significantly reduce your consumption in these situations, which would mean substantially fewer calories taken in.

Treats can be great and there is no reason why you shouldn't have a treat now and then, but it is about getting a good balance and making each one a treat rather than a regular occurrence. Does the twelfth piece of chocolate taste as good as the first? Does the third helping of cake taste as good as the first? Usually the answer is no. Try to make treats small and for special occasions only, and that way you will reduce your overall calorie intake significantly.

Celebrations can be great for you, whether that's your own celebrations, like a birthday or anniversary, or for someone else, such as a wedding, a leaving party, a hen do or a house-warming. But be careful about overindulging unnecessarily on these occasions. If you take some time to consider the calorie and weight-loss equation then you can still have fun, have some treats, enjoy yourself, etc., yet consume much less on the calorie front. With a little motivation, effort and thought you really can make a big difference to your weight.

Cutting out the sugar!

It has been shown how dangerous and addictive sugar can be and how you are likely to find it in many more places than you might think in terms of your food and drink consumption. So how can you cut out the sugar or at least reduce it substantially? The average daily amount of sugar recommended for an adult is around 60 grams, which equates to 15 teaspoons, and most people far exceed this amount.

Firstly it is really important to understand how much sugar you do have, so try to calculate this over a period of say a week and average it out to get a daily figure. Make sure you include all sugar in its many forms and from all food and drink products you consume. You may be surprised how much sugar there is in so-called 'healthy' products, particularly 'low-fat' products. It would be normal for low-fat yoghurt to have 20g of sugar and a low-fat muffin to have 35g. Cereals and cereal bars are another source of large amounts of sugar, although they are perceived to be healthy, as are other foods like baked beans and salad dressings.

Soft drinks, energy drinks, flavoured water, iced coffees and milkshakes will also usually contain large amounts of sugar as do fruit juices and smoothies. Although fruits contain many healthy nutrients they also contain a lot of sugar in the form of fructose.

Make a real effort to be sugar aware and then to cut right back and go for alternative foods and drinks. Try out various techniques that may work for you if you get a sugar craving – go for a quick few minutes' workout, for example, a dance, a fast walk, run up and down the stairs. This can quickly reduce the craving and take your mind off the sugar! Or go for a healthy herbal tea or chew some sugar-free gum. Get into a habit of alternative food and drink options and the more you can do this the easier it will become. You will get fewer cravings and the sugar reduction will become more straightforward; as a result you will have more energy, be in a better mood and lose weight.

Grow your own fruit and vegetables

An excellent way to eat more healthily and lose weight if needed is to grow your own fruit and vegetables. If you have a garden then there is no reason why you can't have a go at growing some different fruits and vegetables and even if you don't have a garden you may be able to find a nearby allotment or a friend, relative or neighbour who is happy for you to use their garden.

Apart from the actual fruit and vegetables, there is a good chance the work will help you, too, through being outside in the fresh air and sunlight, and in the exercise and activity involved with producing, growing and looking after them. And of course the fruit and vegetables will be very good for you, especially in their untampered, organic, fresh, home-grown condition.

If you have children this is a great way to get them involved, interested and excited by fruit and vegetables. Having them help plant, cultivate and pick the different foods is much more likely to then mean they will eat, and thus benefit from, these fruits and vegetables. They could help cook with them too. Growing your own is also a relatively cheap activity, as well as being healthy and beneficial in many ways, so if you can then give it a go and involve others too.

Exercise and activity

We all know that exercise and physical activity are good for us and helps us to burn calories, so they can be a major factor with regard to weight loss. Many people may not be very physically active and could be intimidated or scared of going to the gym or feeling unable to run or take part in various sports or activities. If this is the case then there are still so many activities and forms of exercise that can be done which will be beneficial and help with weight loss.

Another book in this series that I would recommend you read is called *The Real Benefits of Exercise*. It goes into much more detail about exercise and physical activity for people at all levels. If you are unfit, or a beginner when it comes to exercise, then make sure you build up slowly and sensibly and find activities that you can do, will benefit from and will continue with. There are so many options, and anything you do will increase your calorie burning and your metabolism.

Look to involve supportive and encouraging friends, sign up to classes and group activities if you can, ask for expert advice if possible, and also make sure you warm up, cool down and stretch appropriately to help avoid any potential injuries. And try to make exercise and activities part of your lifestyle rather than an extra chore that you grudgingly fit in. It can be fun, exciting, interesting and something you look forward to, and the more options you explore in order to find those exercises and classes that you enjoy, the better. Exercise is very good for you in lots of ways, not just in losing weight.

Be sensible and careful with your food and drink intake with regard to the added exercise. Most importantly be aware of the weight-loss equation of calories in and calories out. Do not eat and drink extra to replace all the extra calories burned through exercise, because you want your body to burn the excess fat you are carrying. Be sensible with what and when you eat and drink. Generally, you will actually feel more energised the more exercise you do, too.

Good food types

In the Healthy Eating section of this book there is much more detail and information on different food types and their effect. Most people will have a basic knowledge and understanding of what is good and what is bad for them but perhaps they will not appreciate the consequences or scale of the potential health problems that can result from eating the wrong food. The more knowledge you have the more likely you are to have a healthy food intake and make the healthier choices, thus improving your health and reducing the potential risks of poor diet and being overweight.

Generally speaking you can eat as many salads and vegetables as you like as they are low-calorie, contain mainly vital nutrients, provide energy and have very little unhealthy sugar and fats. There are so many to choose from and here are just some examples:

Cucumber, tomatoes, lettuce, rocket, spinach, celery, peppers, cabbage, carrots, onions, radishes, sweetcorn, peas, mangetout, French beans, broccoli, cauliflower, courgettes, bean sprouts, aubergines, marrow and asparagus. (I'm sure you can think of more!)

Protein is also important for many reasons, and meat and fish can be a very good source of protein, though try to have lean meat rather than fatty and processed meat products. Beans and pulses such as lentils, kidney beans, broad beans, butter beans and chickpeas can be a good non-meat protein food type. Dairy products like milk, yoghurt and cheese can be good sources of protein but may also be high in fat, so again be careful.

Try to cut out as many processed foods as possible, as they will usually contain a lot of salt, sugars, preservatives and additives with much less nutritional value and higher calorie content. They may be convenient but they are not healthy. The more natural, raw, untouched foods the better. Go for the more colourful and attractive foods rather than the dull, beige, manufactured stuff that is unfortunately so common.

And become more inquisitive and knowledgeable about food and drink labelling. Make an effort to look at the ingredients and breakdown of sugars, salts, fats, proteins, carbohydrates, etc., and don't be fooled by the advertising and marketing of most products.

The right times to eat

We all need to eat and for most of us eating can be very enjoyable as well as necessary. However, apart from what we eat and how much we eat there can be another factor that influences our health and wellbeing, and that is when we eat.

Many people will form eating habits (when and how often they eat) that are not particularly good and have adverse effects. For example, many people will skip breakfast, which can cause poor eating habits later in the day as a result. They may lack energy and possibly experience a lowering of mood, as well as the body then craving more food to compensate, so they may binge eat or snack more and be attracted to the more unhealthy sugar-rich foods and drinks. Skipping breakfast regularly will also cause the body to store additional fat to compensate.

The human body is generally very good at regulating its food intake and digesting well through the course of a day so that it is very possible to have just three well-balanced meals per day – breakfast, lunch and dinner. There is no need to snack or eat between meals if they are nutritious, well-balanced and the right size portions, and you won't feel hungry or have cravings. However, because many people do not eat healthy, well-balanced meals and get into poor habits they tend to eat quite a lot of snacks and additional foods and drinks during the day. A poor diet will also make you lethargic and lower your mood so the temptation to counter this with a snack or a treat to pick you up is often great, and unhealthy snacks are usually readily available.

If you eat a good healthy breakfast and lunch you will be more energised and your blood sugar-levels more consistent meaning you will not feel so hungry and crave the unhealthy foods as much. If you don't eat well in the morning and during the day you will more likely eat a lot more later in the day, in the evenings and into the night as the cravings get stronger. Eating more at this time of day is very likely to mean you will put on weight because you won't be burning off the excess calories, and it could affect your sleep, thus contributing further to the cycle of feeling tired and eating high-sugar foods and putting on weight.

Portion sizes

There is no doubt that in general our portion sizes are far larger than they need to be, and if we decreased our portion sizes on a regular basis a lot less food would be consumed and then a lot of weight would be lost. This is particularly the case when we eat out, get takeaways or cook family-style meals at home. There are many reasons why our portion sizes are so large, but none of them should prevent you from being able to reduce your portion sizes.

The brain and body still behave as if they are unsure when the next meal will be available and so will naturally want to eat as much as possible and then store reserves for emergencies, as this was what was necessary for hundreds of thousands of years as humans evolved. However, this is no longer the case and we shouldn't tempt our brain and body with more food than they need. If you have a larger-than-needed portion size it will be very difficult not to eat it, because this goes against human instincts, so you must take responsibility and stick to smaller sizes.

There is also a temptation to get your money's worth wherever possible and that inevitably means eating (and drinking) as much as possible with the 'all you can eat' buffets, or the bargain offer if you 'go large' or on the all-inclusive holiday deals. Before thinking of the immediate financial benefits to any deals or offers, think about your health and the future cost of being overweight and unhealthy.

At home consider your portion sizes, the size of your plates and what is necessary rather than what you have always done. Simply by cutting down on your portion sizes you can reduce your calorie intake and lose weight. If you can get into the habit of eating less this way it will become easier and feel much more normal, and you will see and feel results.

There is even evidence that suggests the colour of your plates can make a difference! If you have white/cream plates then you will generally have larger portions of those coloured type foods e.g. pasta, rice, potatoes, etc., which are more likely to add to your weight. And if your plates are more colourful you will have less of those types of foods and more of the healthier, more colourful vegetables!

Weight loss for children

Unfortunately there is a growing trend of children becoming overweight and obese. The rates are increasing and the age at which these weight problems are occurring is continuing to get lower, which is worrying for a number of reasons and is only going to lead to more health problems, more strains on our health services and more costs to our society. It is so important to tackle this problem and this starts with education.

We must educate children, with greater responsibility placed on parents, schools and governments, so that children understand food better and realise the benefits of exercise and the dangers of being overweight. The more knowledge and understanding they have the more likely the healthier choices will be made and better habits formed.

It is possible to make this education fun and interesting and more engaging in lots of ways, teaching them all the benefits of a healthy lifestyle and all the risks and dangers of an unhealthy lifestyle. Reward, praise and recognise healthy behaviour and actions so they want to do more. Invest time, effort and money in this as the benefits to their health and happiness are worth it.

Too often adults take the easier, quicker options of fast food, bribing children with sweets and other unhealthy 'treats' and allowing them to sit in front of a computer screen or TV for hours on end. Of course, it can be hard work, tiring and stressful looking after children, but there is also a responsibility to take care of them and that includes looking after their health and happiness and making more of the right choices in this respect.

Nearly all young children will naturally run about, be active, want to play and only eat when they are hungry. Keep encouraging this activity, exercise and play. Experiment with a range of different healthy foods and drinks and encourage them to learn about ingredients and what is good and bad for them. As a result of an improved diet and more exercise they are far more likely to sleep better, work harder, be happier, do well at school, laugh more, make more friends and overall be much healthier, which should continue as they develop and mature into adults.

Make it a lifestyle

It is far easier to improve and maintain your health and happiness if it becomes a lifestyle. If you make the healthy choices regularly and keep practising these, they become 'normal' and you form good habits that are both sustainable and easier to stick to. Otherwise these choices can become a burden or hard work, which requires much more effort and is more likely to fail.

Smaller portion sizes, less sugar, fewer processed foods, more vegetables and salad, more exercise and activity, being more knowledgeable, checking ingredients, investing in your sleep, etc., are all examples of things you can do to improve your health as part of your lifestyle; the more of this you do the easier it becomes and the greater the benefits.

Don't let other people influence you in a bad way and don't be tempted by unhealthy bargains, special offers and promotions. Remember you are what you eat and you are meant to be active so eat the good things and do more exercise and you will feel so much better, which then has a massive positive knock-on effect on all aspects of your life.

Eat Healthy! Feel Healthy! Be Healthy!

Part 2

Healthy Eating

'I really regret eating healthily today'... said no one ever!

Introduction

In order to improve your health directly through what you eat and drink it is important to understand more about the different types of food, what they are for and what their effects are on both body and mind, and to look more closely at labelling on products and understand what the numbers and words mean. This section aims to provide that information, and don't forget the all-important saying 'you are what you eat'.

So being more aware of what you consume and what is healthy and unhealthy will mean you are more likely to become a healthier eater and be able to educate others, too, so not just you becoming healthier and happier as a result!

'Let your food be your medicine and your medicine be your food.' – Hippocrates

Understanding Food

Understanding calories

Calories are a measure of the amount of energy in food. Knowing how many calories are in our food can help us to balance the energy we put into our bodies with the energy we use. And that's the key to a healthy weight.

An average man needs around 2,500kcal (10,500kJ) a day. For an average woman, that figure is around 2,000kcal (8,400kJ). These values can vary depending on age and levels of physical activity, among other factors

We measure the amount of energy contained in an item of food in calories, just as we measure the weight of that item of food in kilograms. If you're trying to lose weight, it's a good idea to eat less and be more active. Eating less is important when you're trying to lose weight, even if you already have a balanced diet.

Calories and energy balance

When we eat and drink, we're putting energy (calories) into our bodies. Our bodies then use up that energy, and the more physical activity we do, the more energy (calories) we use.

To maintain a stable weight, the energy we put into our bodies must be the same as the energy we use for normal bodily functions and physical activity. If there are some days where we put in more energy than we use, then there should also be days where the opposite is true, so that overall the energy in and energy used remain balanced.

Weight gain occurs when we regularly put more energy into our bodies than we use. Over time, that excess energy is stored by the body as fat. Research shows that most adults eat and drink more than they need, and also think that they are more physically active than they are.

Checking calories in food

Knowing the calorie content of foods can be a useful tool when it comes to achieving or maintaining a healthy weight. It can help us to keep track of the amount of energy we are eating and drinking, and ensure we're not consuming too much.

The calorie content of many foods is stated in the nutrition label, which you will often find on the back or side of the packaging. This information will appear under the 'Energy' heading. The calorie content is often given in kcals, which is short for kilocalories, and also in kJ, which is short for kilojoules.

Calorie counters

There is a wide range of online calorie counters. We can't verify their data but they can help you track your calories. Examples include:

- My Meal Mate
- MyFitnessPal
- Calorie counting
- FatSecret

A 'kilocalorie' is another word for what is commonly called a 'calorie', so 1,000 calories will be written as 1,000kcals. Kilojoules are the metric measurement of calories. To find the energy content in kilojoules, multiply the calorie figure by 4.2.

The label will usually tell you how many calories are contained in 100g or 100ml of the food or drink, so you can compare the calorie content of different products. Many labels will also state the number of calories in 'one portion' of the food. But remember that the manufacturer's idea of 'one portion' may not be the same as yours, so there could be more calories in the portion you serve yourself.

You can use the calorie information to assess how a particular food fits into your daily calorie intake. As a guide, remember the average man needs 2,500kcal (10,500kJ) to maintain his weight, and the average woman needs 2,000kcal (8,400kJ). Some restaurants put calorie information on their menus, so you can also check calorie content of foods when eating out. Calories should be given per portion or per meal.

Checking the calories you use

The number of calories people use by doing a particular physical activity varies depending on a range of factors, including size and age. The more vigorously you do an activity, the more calories you will use. For example, fast walking will use more calories than walking at a moderate pace.

Losing weight

If you're gaining weight, it usually means you've been regularly eating and drinking more calories than you've been using through normal bodily functions and physical activity. To lose weight you have to tip that balance in the other direction; you must start to use more energy than you consume, and do this over a sustained period of time.

You can do this by making healthy changes to your diet so that you eat and drink fewer calories. The best approach is to combine these changes with increased physical activity. You can also talk to your GP or practice nurse and get more advice on achieving the right energy balance and losing weight.

Understanding fats

We all need some fat in our diet. But too much of a particular kind of fat – saturated fat – can raise our cholesterol, which increases the risk of heart disease. It's important to cut down on fat and choose foods that contain unsaturated fat.

Eating too much fat can also make us more likely to put on weight, because foods that are high in fat are high in energy too, which is measured in kilojoules (kJ) or calories (kcal). Being overweight raises our risk of serious health problems, such as type 2 diabetes and high blood pressure, as well as coronary heart disease.

But this doesn't mean that all fat is bad. We need some fat in our diet because it helps the body absorb certain nutrients. Fat is a source of energy as well as some vitamins (such as vitamins A and D), and provides essential fatty acids that the body can't make itself.

There are two main types of fat found in food: saturated and unsaturated. But which fats should we be eating more of?

As part of a healthy diet, we should try to cut down on food that is high in **saturated fat**.

Saturated fat

Most people in the UK eat too much saturated fat: about 20% more than the recommended maximum, according to the British Dietetic Association.

- The average man should eat no more than 30g of saturated fat a day.

- The average woman should eat no more than 20g of saturated fat a day.

Eating a diet high in saturated fat can cause the level of cholesterol in your blood to build up over time. Raised cholesterol increases your risk of heart disease.

Foods high in saturated fat include:

- fatty cuts of meat
- meat products, including sausages and pies
- butter and lard
- cheese, especially hard cheese
- cream, soured cream and ice cream
- some savoury snacks and chocolate confectionery
- biscuits, cakes and pastries

Trans fats

Trans fats are found naturally at low levels in some foods, such as those from animals, including meat and dairy products. They can also be found in foods containing hydrogenated vegetable oil.

Hydrogenated vegetable oils may contain trans fats. If a food contains hydrogenated vegetable oil then this must be declared on the ingredients list.

Like saturated fats, trans fats can raise cholesterol levels in the blood. This is why it's recommended that trans fats should make up no more than 2% of the energy (kJ/kcal) we get from our diet. For adults, this is no more than about 5g a day.

However, most people in the UK don't eat a lot of trans fats. On average, we eat about half the recommended maximum. Most of the supermarkets in the UK have removed hydrogenated vegetable oil from all their own-brand products. We eat a lot more saturated fats than trans fats. This means that when looking at the amount of fat in your diet, it's more important to focus on reducing the amount of saturated fat.

Remember, we don't need to cut down on every type of fat. Some fats are not only good for us, most people should be eating more of them.

Unsaturated fats

Eating unsaturated fats instead of saturated can help lower blood cholesterol. Unsaturated fat, such as omega-3 essential fatty acids, is found in:

- oily fish such as salmon, sardines and mackerel
- nuts and seeds
- sunflower and olive oils

Unsaturated fats are also found in some fruit and vegetables, such as avocados.

Nutrition labels on food packaging can help you to reduce the amount of fat you eat:

High-fat foods: more than 17.5g of total fat per 100g

Low-fat foods: less than 3g of total fat per 100g

These tips can help you cut the total amount of fat in your diet:

- **Compare nutrition labels when shopping**, so you can pick foods lower in fat. Use the 'per serving' or 'per 100g' information to compare different foods. Remember, servings may vary, so read the label carefully.

- **Ask your butcher for lean cuts of meat**, or compare nutrition labels on meat packaging.

- **Choose lower-fat dairy products**, such as 1% fat milk or lower-fat cheese.

- **Grill, bake, poach or steam food** rather than frying or roasting, so that you won't need to add any extra fat.

- **Trim visible fat** and take skin off meat before cooking.

- **Use the grill instead of the frying pan**, whatever meat you're cooking.

- **Put more vegetables or beans in casseroles, stews and curries**, and a bit less meat. And skim the fat off the top before serving.

- **When making sandwiches, try leaving out the butter or spread**: you might not need it if you're using a moist filling. When you do use spread, go for a reduced-fat variety and choose one that is soft straight from the fridge, so it's easier to spread thinly.

Nutrition labels

The nutrition labels on food packaging can help you to cut down on total fat and saturated fat. Labels containing nutrition information are usually on the back of food packaging; they will often tell you how much fat and saturated fat is contained in 100g of the food, and sometimes the amount per portion or per serving.

Some packaging also displays nutrition labels on the front, which give at-a-glance information on specific nutrients. These labels may contain information on recommended daily intakes or colour-coded nutrition information to help you make healthier choices.

When colour-coding is used on food labels, red means 'high'. Leave red foods for the occasional treat, and aim to eat mainly foods that are green or amber.

Total fat

So what counts as high fat and low fat?

- **High**: more than 17.5g of fat per 100g. May be colour-coded red.
- **Low**: 3g of fat or less per 100g. May be colour-coded green.

Saturated fat

Look out for 'saturates' or 'sat fat' on the label: this tells you how much saturated fat is in the food.

- **High:** more than 5g saturates per 100g. May be colour-coded red.
- **Low:** 1.5g saturates or less per 100g. May be colour-coded green.

If the amount of fat or saturated fat per 100g is in between these figures, that's a medium level, and may be colour-coded amber.

What 'lower fat' or 'reduced fat' really means

Just because a food packet contains the words 'lower fat' or 'reduced fat' doesn't necessarily mean it's a healthy choice. The lower-fat claim simply means that the food is 30% lower in fat than the standard equivalent. So if the type of food in question is high in fat in the first place, the lower-fat version may also still be high in fat. For example, a lower-fat mayonnaise is 30% lower in fat than the standard version, but is still high in fat.

Also, these foods aren't necessarily low in calories. Often the fat is replaced with sugar, and the food may end up with the same, or an even higher, energy content. To be sure of the fat content and the energy content, remember to check the nutrition label on the packet. Be very careful about how much sugar is in anything claiming to be low-fat!

Understanding salt

Salt is a chemical called sodium chloride and we commonly recognise it as the small white crystals that we shake onto our food. However, most of the salt you eat isn't what you add to food yourself, as most salt is hidden in the processed foods you consume. Takeaway and restaurant foods are also often high in salt. It's even found in foods where you might not expect to find it, such as cakes and biscuits, bread and breakfast cereals.

The two components of salt, sodium and chloride, are both important for several processes within your body. Sodium is essential for your nerves to work properly and for you to be able to contract your muscles. Chloride is an important part of the juices in your stomach and bowels and helps you to digest food. Both sodium and chloride help to keep the fluid levels in your body balanced.

A diet high in sodium can increase your risk of developing high blood pressure and if you have too much sodium in your blood, your body will start to hold onto water to try to dilute the sodium. This will increase the amount of fluid in your body and your blood will increase in volume. As this happens, more pressure is put on your blood vessels and your heart has to work harder. Over time, the extra pressure and work can stiffen your blood vessels and cause high blood pressure. If you have high blood pressure, you're more likely to get several major illnesses, including heart disease and stroke and it may also lead to heart failure.

You do need a small amount of salt in your diet, with the recommended amount no more than 6g a day, which is just over one teaspoon and equates to roughly 2.3g of sodium a day. It's difficult to eat too little salt; most people eat too much and need to cut down.

Children should have less salt than adults, so don't add any salt to your child's food. Babies should only have a very small amount of salt, because their kidneys can't cope with much. When your baby starts to eat solid foods, don't add salt to any foods that you prepare for him or her. Also, remember not to give your child foods that aren't specifically suitable for babies, as these may be high in salt.

When you buy food products, check the label and see how much salt is in a product per 100g. Anything with over 1.5g is high in salt, so only eat these foods occasionally. Foods with 0.3g or less of salt are generally a healthy choice. Compare labels when you're shopping and choose products that are lower in salt. Not all labels will tell you the salt content of a product. Some will tell you the amount of sodium instead. You can work out the amount of salt by multiplying the sodium content by 2.5.

Finally, try not to add too much extra salt to your food. It may be hard at first, but if you reduce the amount of salt you use gradually, you will get used to having less salt and you may start to enjoy the taste of your food more.

To help cut down on your salt intake try these tips:

- Cut down on processed foods, as these contain a lot of salt – eat fresh foods wherever possible.

- Experiment with garlic, pepper, herbs and spices or a squeeze of lemon to flavour your food, instead of salt.

- Taste your food before you add salt at the table – it might already be tasty enough without adding salt.

- Pick canned vegetables and pulses such as baked beans that have 'no added salt' on the label.

- Watch out for sauces that can be high in salt, such as tomato ketchup and pasta sauces – choose lower-salt versions where possible.

Understanding carbohydrates

Carbohydrates are compounds that your body uses for energy. They are found in almost every type of food you eat albeit in different forms and amounts. All carbohydrates are made up of individual 'building blocks' or sugar molecules. The most basic carbohydrates such as the sugar you put in your tea, or that gives your apple its sweet taste, consist of just one or two of these molecules.

Other more complex (or 'starchy') carbohydrates are made up of sometimes hundreds of sugar molecules joined together. These are the types of carbohydrate found in bread, pasta and rice, as well as some fruit and vegetables. Fibre is also classed as a carbohydrate. However, unlike other types of carbohydrate, it isn't usually used by your body for energy but has a number of other important functions.

Carbohydrates are your body's main source of energy. You use them as fuel, not only to help you walk or run, but also to keep your heart, lungs and other vital organs working properly. When you eat any type of carbohydrate, your digestive system will break it down into simple sugars, such as glucose – the main form of fuel for your body. Glucose is then circulated in your blood to every cell in your body.

If you don't have enough carbohydrates in your diet, your body will start to break down fat and then protein to get the glucose it needs. Protein is important for your body to be able to grow and repair itself, so using it as an energy source means there will be little left to carry out these vital functions. If you eat enough carbohydrates, you can prevent this.

There has been much misconception in recent times that carbohydrates are fattening. Of course, as with many things, it's not good to have too much. If you eat more carbohydrates than your body can burn off as energy, your body's glucose stores will become saturated and the excess will be converted to fat. In other words, you will start to put on weight. But carbohydrates are an essential part of a healthy diet. The key thing is to pick the right type of carbohydrates, as some are healthier than others.

Foods and drinks that are high in sugar are a major cause of tooth decay. Sugary foods such as cakes and biscuits also tend to be high in fat, but they often don't contain many other useful nutrients – hence the term 'empty calories'. They contribute to your energy intake but have little other value. Not only that, sugary foods are often very energy dense, which means they pack a lot of calories into a small volume. Even if you eat just small amounts of these foods, they can push up your calorie intake. It's therefore best to limit your intake of sugary foods and stick to starchy foods.

In general, the best starchy carbohydrates to go for are wholegrain foods including wholegrain varieties of breads, pasta and cereal. Whole grains contain a host of important nutrients that are thought to reduce your risk of heart disease and bowel cancer. When grains are processed (or 'refined') to make them look whiter, the part of the grain that contains fibre and many useful nutrients is removed. This means that white bread, pasta and cereals aren't as beneficial to your health.

Whole grains are also more likely to keep you feeling fuller for longer as they generally take longer to digest than foods that have been processed, and contain more fibre. This can help to control your appetite and help you to maintain a healthy weight.

It's thought that at least half the energy in your diet should come from carbohydrates. Many people are already eating enough, but it's often the wrong type, with too much coming from sugary or refined products and not enough from wholegrain, starchy foods. Starchy foods should make up about a third of your diet and you should opt for whole grains when possible.

Although it's best to limit the sugar in your diet, this doesn't mean cutting out fruit. The natural sugars in fruit are not as bad for your teeth as those in sugary foods and drinks, as they are held inside the cells of the fruit and only released when you chew it, or if the fruit is juiced or blended in fruit juices and smoothies. If you drink these, try to stick to one a day and drink them with a meal to reduce your risk of tooth decay.

Understanding proteins

Proteins are complex substances, made up of chains of amino acids. Amino acids are building blocks that combine in different formations to make up the proteins in your body. There are 20 amino acids in total and although your body can make some of these itself there are nine that you can only get from protein that you eat. These are called the essential amino acids.

When you eat protein, it's broken down into amino acids. These can then be rearranged into new proteins that your body needs. Protein is essential for the healthy growth of all of your body tissues such as your muscles (including your heart), internal organs (such as your lungs and liver) and skin, and also for repair of these tissues. In addition, it's a good source of energy too.

Different foods contain different amounts of amino acids. Foods that are high in protein are said to be either complete or incomplete proteins. Complete proteins contain all the essential amino acids, whereas incomplete proteins contain some but not all of them.

On the whole, you can only get complete proteins from animal products, such as meat, fish, dairy produce and eggs. The only plant proteins that contain all the essential amino acids are soya beans and foods made from them, and a grain called quinoa. Examples of incomplete proteins include beans and other pulses, nuts and seeds and cereals. However, most people with a balanced diet will eat a wide enough range of foods that contain protein so even if you're a vegetarian, you're likely to be getting all the amino acids your body needs.

Understanding fibre

Fibre is only found in foods from plants, such as beans, grains, vegetables and fruits. It passes through the body with very little change in the digestive system. That means that fibre provides few or no calories, in addition to having many health benefits.

Fibre provides many benefits. While maintaining the health of the digestive tract, it also lowers the risk of certain cancers, heart disease and diabetes. It helps control the appetite, so it's easier to keep weight in check and because it is found only in plant foods, vegetarians tend to have very high fibre intakes, which may be one of the reasons vegetarians are generally healthier and slimmer than meat-eaters.

Health Benefits of Fibre

- **Colon and rectal cancer:** Increasing fibre can help decrease the risk of colon and rectal cancers.

- **Diabetes:** Diets high in fibre help control blood-sugar levels and have also been shown to decrease the risk of developing type 2 diabetes.

- **Heart disease:** Fibre can reduce blood-cholesterol levels. Diets high in fibre have also been shown to decrease the risk of heart disease.

- **Diverticulitis:** Fibre decreases the risk of diverticulitis, a painful intestinal condition.

- **Constipation:** Fibre helps prevent constipation.

- **Weight control:** Fibre is filling, has almost no calories, and helps maintain blood sugar – all factors that help control hunger and body weight.

Fibre is an important part of a healthy diet, and a diet high in fibre has many health benefits. It can help prevent heart disease, diabetes, weight gain and some cancers, and can also improve digestive health. However, many people don't get enough fibre. On average, most people in the UK get about 14g of fibre a day. You should aim for at least 18g a day. Fibre is only found in foods that come from plants; foods such as meat, fish and dairy products don't contain any fibre.

There are two different types of fibre – soluble and insoluble. Each type of fibre helps your body in different ways, so a normal, healthy diet should include both types. However, if you have a digestive disorder such as irritable bowel syndrome (IBS), you may need to modify the type and amount of fibre in your diet in accordance with your symptoms. Your GP or a dietitian will be able to advise you further about this.

Soluble fibre

Soluble fibre can be digested by your body. It may help reduce the amount of cholesterol in your blood. If you have constipation, gradually increasing sources of soluble fibre such as fruit and vegetables, oats and golden linseeds can help soften your stools and make them easier to pass.

Foods that contain soluble fibre include:

- oats, barley and rye
- fruit, such as bananas and apples
- root vegetables, such as carrots and potatoes
- golden linseeds

Insoluble fibre

Insoluble fibre can't be digested. It passes through your gut without being broken down and helps other foods move through your digestive system more easily. Insoluble fibre keeps your bowels healthy and helps prevent digestive problems. If you have diarrhoea, you should limit the amount of insoluble fibre in your diet.

Good sources of insoluble fibre include:

- wholemeal bread
- bran
- cereals
- nuts and seeds

Eating foods high in fibre will help you feel fuller for longer and this may help if you are trying to lose weight. If you need to increase your fibre intake, it's important that you do so gradually. A sudden increase may make you produce more wind (flatulence), leave you feeling bloated and cause stomach cramps. It's also important to make sure you drink plenty of fluid. You should drink at least eight glasses of fluid a day, or more while exercising or when it's hot.

Understanding vitamins and minerals

Vitamins and minerals are nutrients that you need in small amounts in order for your body to function properly, and are all found in different foods. There are many different vitamins and minerals and they do different things; some help your body to digest food, for example, and others build strong bones.

What are vitamins?

There are two types of vitamins:

- water-soluble vitamins – you can't store these in your body so you need to get them from your diet
- fat-soluble vitamins – you can store these in your body but they should still be part of a healthy diet

Water-soluble vitamins (such as vitamins B6, B12, C and folic acid) are found in fresh fruit and green vegetables. It's best to eat these foods raw, steamed or grilled rather than boiled because cooking can easily destroy the vitamins.

Fat-soluble vitamins (such as vitamins A, D and E) are mainly found in fatty foods, such as animal fats (including butter and lard), vegetable oils, dairy foods and oily fish.

What are minerals and trace elements?

Your body needs small amounts of minerals and trace elements in order to function properly. They are as essential as vitamins and your body has to get them from the food you eat. For example, you need:

- calcium to make strong bones
- sodium to balance the fluids in your body and to help nerves function
- iron to help your body transport oxygen in your blood and to break down and release energy from the food you eat

You can find minerals and trace elements in meat, cereals, fish, dairy foods, vegetables, dried fruit and nuts.

How much do I need?

The amount of vitamins and minerals your body needs is individual to you and varies from person to person. It can depend on many things, including your gender, age and activity levels.

The Department of Health gives guidance on the levels of nutrients to have in your diet, although these aren't exact recommendations. They are called dietary reference values and you will usually find them listed on food and supplement packets. These values show how much of a particular nutrient a group of people of a certain age range (and sometimes gender) need for good health.

How can I get enough vitamins and minerals?

Most people are able to get most of the vitamins and minerals they need by eating a healthy, balanced diet. Aim to eat at least five servings of fruit and vegetables each day. It's important to include starchy foods (such as bread, potatoes and pasta) and moderate amounts of protein-rich foods (such as meat, fish and pulses) in your meals.

Vitamin D is the one vitamin you can't get from diet alone. It's in foods such as oily fish, but only in small amounts. Vitamin D is produced naturally by your body when your skin is exposed to sunlight. You may get enough vitamin D during summer by spending frequent short spells in the sun without wearing sunscreen (the exact time you need is different for everyone, but is typically only a few minutes in the middle of the day). However, don't let your skin burn. For more information about safety in the sun, see our factsheet, Sun care. Certain people can be at risk of vitamin D deficiency, including those who are over 65 and don't get out in the sun much, or women who are pregnant. If you're concerned that you may not be getting enough vitamin D, ask your GP for advice.

What about supplements?

If you eat a healthy, balanced diet, it will supply most of the vitamins you need. You will only need to take supplements if your GP recommends you do so. Your GP may advise you to take supplements if you're planning a pregnancy for example, and need extra folic acid. You may also need to take supplements if you're at risk of osteoporosis and need vitamin D and calcium, or if you have age-related macular degeneration and need supplements of vitamins C, E and zinc. However, it's important to get advice, as some vitamin supplements (containing vitamins A and E) may be harmful.

If you don't get much sun exposure and particularly during winter months, taking up to 25 micrograms of vitamin D a day (two high-strength 12.5 microgram capsules) can help to make sure you get enough.

Always read the patient information leaflet that comes with your supplements and if you are pregnant or breastfeeding, ask your pharmacist or GP for advice first. Talk to your GP before taking vitamin D supplements if you are taking diuretics for high blood pressure or have a history of kidney stones or kidney failure

Adapting your diet

There will be times during your life when you need to adapt your diet to suit your changing needs. For example, if you become pregnant or simply as you get older. Likewise if you decide to become vegetarian or vegan you may have to rethink your diet to make sure you get all the nutrients you need.

People over 50

As you get older it's especially important to eat plenty of iron-rich foods to stay healthy. This will lower your risk of developing iron-deficiency anaemia, which can make you feel tired and weaken your immune system. Iron is in a range of foods, including red meat, fish such as sardines, eggs, pulses, fortified breakfast cereals and green leafy vegetables.

Caffeine interferes with your body's ability to absorb iron and other nutrients. So although you may feel you can't function without your morning cup, if you think you're not getting enough iron, try not to have tea or coffee with, or immediately after, your breakfast, or any other meal. Drink fruit juice instead as this will help your body to absorb iron. Aim to eat five servings of fruit and vegetables each day to keep your immune system healthy.

Osteoporosis is a major health issue for older people, particularly women, so it's vital to have plenty of calcium. Dairy products, such as milk, cheese and yoghurt, are excellent sources of calcium as is fish with bones, such as pilchards or sardines. As with calcium, vitamin D is important for good bone health too. You get most of your vitamin D from the effect of sunlight on your skin but you can also get it from your diet in oily fish and eggs, for example. If you're over 65, or are housebound, your GP may recommend you take vitamin D supplements.

If you think you may need a vitamin or mineral supplement, talk to your GP. He or she will check that you take the right dose and ensure the supplements don't affect any medicines you're taking.

Pregnant women

There is a lot to think about when you get pregnant but one key thing to remember is to eat properly. Eat a healthy, balanced diet and make sure you get enough iron as your body's supply can drop when you're pregnant. It's also important to eat plenty of foliate-rich foods (foliate is the natural form of folic acid). Good sources include broccoli, oranges and wholegrain foods. Eat plenty of dairy foods as this will provide lots of calcium for your baby's growing bones.

As well as eating a healthy diet, the UK Department of Health recommends that women take a 400-microgram folic acid supplement while trying for a baby and during the first three months of pregnancy. This will help to reduce your baby's risk of spina bifida and other neural tube defects. The Department of Health also suggests you take a 10-microgram vitamin D supplement while pregnant and if you're breastfeeding. They also recommend that babies and children take a vitamin D supplement up to the age of five.

Vegetarians and vegans

It's perfectly possible to get all the vitamins and minerals you need from a vegetarian diet. Aim to:

- eat five servings of fruit and vegetables every day

- eat plenty of iron-rich foods (such as green vegetables and fortified breakfast cereals)

- base your meals on starchy foods (such as bread, rice and pasta) and a good source of protein (such as dairy or soya products, pulses and nuts)

- keep up your level of calcium – if you don't drink cows' milk, choose soya, rice or oat drinks fortified with calcium

- ensure you get a good supply of vitamin B12 by eating fortified cereals or yeast extract

Vegetables and salads

Vegetables and salads should be seen as the REAL comfort foods, with nutrients that actually improve your resilience to stress. Eating vegetables helps replenish your magnesium and vitamin C, which can be depleted by stress. Vegetables also provide you with omega-3 fats and B vitamins, proven to help reduce anxiety and depression. The vitamin K in veggies helps reduce inflammation in your body, which stress can aggravate.

Green leafy vegetables, such as kale and spinach, are loaded with magnesium, which helps balance your cortisol, one of your 'stress hormones'. Magnesium and potassium relax blood vessels, helping keep your blood pressure low. Magnesium also plays an important role in calcium absorption, helping you maintain good muscle and nerve function and a healthy immune system. Low magnesium levels have been linked with anxiety disorders and migraines, both of which are typically aggravated by stress.

Avocados are one of the best stress-busting foods you can eat, replete with potassium, glutathione, healthy fats and more foliate than any other fruit. Asparagus is also rich in foliate, which is extremely important for your brain.

Fresh vegetables are also great when it comes to bone health. They offer high forms of calcium, magnesium, silica, and a host of other minerals that work synergistically to build strong, healthy bones. One of the fat-soluble vitamins playing a critical role in bone health is vitamin K2, as its primary function is to move calcium into the proper areas (teeth and bones). Vitamin K2 also helps direct calcium away from areas where it can cause problems, such as your arteries and soft tissues.

One of the best sources of vitamin K2 is fermented vegetables made with a special starter culture designed to optimise this nutrient. Fennel is also very good for your bones, particularly the seeds. Research has shown that eating the seeds of the fennel plant has a beneficial effect on bone mineral density, as well as bone mineral content. Researchers found that fennel seeds show potential in preventing bone loss in post-menopausal osteoporosis.

Most vegetables and salads are naturally low in fat and calories so are great for losing weight. None have cholesterol. (Though be careful of sauces, dressings or seasonings as they may add fat, sugar, calories or cholesterol.) Vegetables are important sources of many nutrients, including potassium, dietary fibre, foliate (folic acid), vitamin A and vitamin C. Vitamin A keeps eyes and skin healthy and helps to protect against infections. Vitamin C helps heal cuts and wounds, keeps teeth and gums healthy and aids in iron absorption.

Diets rich in potassium may help to maintain healthy blood pressure. Vegetable sources of potassium include sweet potatoes, white potatoes, white beans, tomato products (paste, sauce and juice), beet greens, soybeans, lima beans, spinach, lentils and kidney beans.

Dietary fibre from vegetables, as part of an overall healthy diet, helps reduce blood cholesterol levels and may lower risk of heart disease. Fibre is important for proper bowel function. It helps reduce constipation and diverticulitis. Fibre-containing foods such as vegetables help provide a feeling of fullness with fewer calories.

A great way to eat more vegetables is to store them in your freezer so you always have some to hand and they don't go off or out of date very quickly. Frozen vegetables will keep their nutritional value and are just as good as fresh vegetables and are easy to prepare from frozen. So stock up that freezer with healthy vegetables!

Understanding processed foods

Processed foods aren't just microwave meals and other ready meals. The term 'processed food' applies to any food that has been altered from its natural state in some way and this means you are probably eating more processed food than you realise. Although processed foods aren't necessarily unhealthy, anything that's been processed is much more likely to contain added salt, sugar and fat.

Another benefit of cooking food from scratch at home or buying natural, raw, unprocessed foods is that you know exactly what is going into it, including the amount of added salt or sugar.

Examples of common processed foods include:

- breakfast cereals
- cheese
- tinned vegetables
- bread
- savoury snacks, such as crisps
- meat products, such as bacon
- 'convenience foods', such as microwave meals or ready meals
- drinks, such as milk or soft drinks

Food processing techniques include freezing, canning, baking, drying and pasteurising products. Not all processed food is a bad choice. Some foods need processing to make them safe, such as milk, which needs to be pasteurised to remove harmful bacteria. Other foods need processing to make them suitable for use, such as pressing seeds to make oil.

Ingredients such as salt, sugar and fat are often added to processed foods to make their flavour more appealing and to prolong their shelf life, or in some cases to contribute to the food's structure. This can lead to people eating more than the recommended amounts for these additives, as they may not be aware of how much has been added to the food they are buying and eating. These foods can also be higher in calories owing to the large amounts of added sugar or fat in them.

Furthermore, a diet high in red and processed meat (regularly eating more than 90g a day) has also been linked to an increased risk of bowel cancer. Some studies have also shown that eating a large amount of processed meat may be linked to a higher risk of cancer or heart disease.

Processed meat refers to meat that has been preserved by smoking, curing, salting or adding preservatives. This includes sausages, bacon, ham, salami and pâtés. The Department of Health recommends that if you currently eat more than 90g (cooked weight) of red and processed meat a day, that you cut down to 70g a day. This is equivalent to two or three rashers of bacon, or a little over two slices of roast lamb, beef or pork.

Other factors

The benefits of water and hydration

Stay slimmer with water

Water can help you to lose weight as it helps you feel full. Try replacing calorie-laden drinks with plain water and drink a glass before meals to help you feel fuller. Drinking more water can help pump up your metabolism, especially if your glass is icy cold. Your body must work to warm the water up, burning a few extra calories in the process.

Water boosts your energy

If you're feeling drained and depleted, get a pick-me-up with water. Dehydration makes you feel fatigued. Water helps the blood transport oxygen and other essential nutrients to your cells. If you're getting enough water, your heart also doesn't have to work as hard to pump blood throughout your body.

Exercise more

Drinking water helps prevent muscle cramping and lubricates joints in the body. When you're well hydrated, you can exercise longer and stronger without 'hitting the wall'. Additionally, being hydrated can prevent headaches and other pains that will be annoying, painful and unpleasant as well as stopping you from being more active.

Nourish your skin

Fine lines and wrinkles are deeper when you're dehydrated. Water is nature's own beauty cream. Drinking water hydrates skin cells and plumps them up, making your face look younger. It also flushes out impurities and improves circulation and blood flow, leaving your face clean, clear and glowing.

Stay regular with water

Along with fibre, water is essential for good digestion. Water helps dissolve waste particles and pass them smoothly through your digestive tract. If you're dehydrated, your body absorbs all the water, leaving your bowel motions dry and more difficult to pass.

Water reduces kidney stones

The rate of painful kidney stones is rising because people, including children, aren't drinking enough water. Water dilutes the salts and minerals in your urine that form the solid crystals known as kidney stones. Kidney stones are less likely to form in diluted urine, so reduce your risk with plenty of water!

Are you drinking enough water?

Generally, nutritionists recommend that you drink eight glasses of water a day though you will need more water if you exercise or sweat heavily. Try to get in the habit of having a water bottle with you and drinking water regularly as a normal part of your day.

Alcohol

Alcohol has a depressant effect on the brain so drinking it can result in a rapid worsening of your mood. It is also a toxin that has to be deactivated by the liver. During this detoxification process the body uses thiamine, zinc and other nutrients and this can deplete your reserves, especially if your diet is poor.

Thiamine and other vitamin deficiencies are common in heavy drinkers and these deficits can cause low mood, irritability and/or aggressive behaviour as well as more serious and long-term mental health problems. Because the body uses important nutrients to manage the processing of alcohol, people who experience depression should consider abstaining from alcohol use until they have recovered. Even then, because of alcohol's depressant effects they should consider drinking only small amounts, perhaps no more than once a week.

There are also a lot of calories in alcohol and alcoholic beverages so be careful and look closely at the label. Many people focus on the calories they consume from food and ignore or forget about the calories from drinks. There are also the additional problems – that drinking alcohol can make you feel more tired, you may get hangovers, your fitness levels are likely to fall and you will be less physically active.

Some people's appetite increases when consuming alcohol so they eat more than necessary, or they crave more unhealthy foods, thus putting on more weight. You will be less inclined to make an effort with your healthy diet if you are drinking alcohol and your motivation to be healthy in general is likely to diminish too.

Food and mood

Your mood can increase and decrease both directly and indirectly as a result of the food you eat. A healthy diet will directly improve your mood, helping to boost and regulate various hormones and neurotransmitters in the brain as well as having a direct benefit to your body, organs and skin. Indirectly you will feel better about yourself as you will be pleased and proud that you have eaten well and been healthy, further improving your mood, confidence and self-esteem. This should also help to maintain or even improve your motivation to eat healthily.

If you eat unhealthily then this too will directly impact your mood, as it negatively affects your brain chemistry and your body, organs and skin. You may get an initial 'high' and better mood from certain unhealthy foods, but when you come down the low is generally worse and will last longer than the high. Feeling lethargic, full, bloated and generally unhealthy will also affect your mood and you are likely to feel worse about yourself for various reasons. A lack of discipline, knowing you shouldn't have eaten that, being ashamed of yourself, beating yourself up about what you have done, etc., are all possible results which are not good and will not benefit you.

Many people will comfort eat for a variety of reasons but most who do this are fully aware it is bad for them and will often feel worse after they have consumed the unhealthy food, so the initial comfort soon fades and is taken over by guilt, shame, a worse mood, being more depressed, etc. The food we consume really does have a huge impact on how we behave, how happy we are, what we do, how we are with others and how we feel about ourselves. In so many ways we are what we eat and therefore if we eat well and in a healthy way then we will feel well and healthy, and of course the opposite is generally true too.

A great idea if you can do it is to record a food and drink diary and alongside it keep a mood diary. Write down what you consume and when and how your mood is throughout a day; do this for a couple of weeks. It is likely you will see some strong correlations between your food and your mood in both a good and a bad way.

Preventing illness

What you eat and drink can also play a big role in preventing and overcoming common illnesses as well as the diseases and health conditions we have already discussed. For example, you can significantly reduce your chances of getting colds and flu if you eat healthily, and if you do get ill then you will deal with it and recover much more quickly. Ensuring your body gets the right vitamins, minerals and nutrients and is not deficient in these can play an important role in maintaining a healthy and active immune system.

You are also less likely to get ulcers, skin problems, rashes, infections, headaches, irritable bowel syndrome, constipation, diarrhoea, coughs and sore throats as examples of illnesses that affect people. With healthy eating and drinking you can directly and indirectly reduce your chances of being affected by these and be able to overcome them more quickly. If your body is healthy – weight good, fitness levels reasonable – and your diet is healthy then your immune system will be working more effectively. Nobody likes being ill and it can cause many additional problems, so reduce your risk and go for the healthy eating!

'Every time you eat or drink, you are either feeding disease or fighting it.'

Cooking healthily

There are many benefits from cooking and especially 'healthy' cooking. There are many reasons or excuses why people tend to cook less and less for themselves these days or spend less time cooking, yet in most cases the benefits of cooking healthily for yourself far outweigh these reasons or excuses if you look at them objectively.

Some of the benefits of cooking for yourself include the fact it is a positive and productive thing to do, which means you can feel satisfied and indeed have a sense of pride and fulfilment for your efforts. You will feel good about yourself as you know that cooking a healthy meal is far better than the many other alternatives of processed foods, microwave foods, takeaways, snacks, fast foods, etc. So emotionally and mentally you will feel better just from the process of cooking your own food and making that effort.

Furthermore, if you are cooking a healthy meal then you are far more likely to use fresher ingredients with fewer additives, preservatives, chemicals, fats, sugars, salts, etc. You will benefit from these cleaner, fresher, more natural, less tampered-with products and ingredients.

People will often mention that healthy food is more expensive; however, I would say that isn't always the case and in fact it is easily possible to eat and cook healthily at low cost and it can be significantly cheaper than many of the alternatives people choose. Also, what price do you put on your health? Let's say you spend an extra £2.50 per day on healthy food but as a result you are much healthier and happier and will live longer!

In addition, the process of buying ingredients, cooking them and then cleaning up all involves being active, which is good for you! It is far better for your health to do that and be active in the process than to pick out a processed ready meal from the freezer and put it in the microwave or ring up your local Chinese takeaway to deliver your food. Plus, the more you cook healthily, the easier it is and it becomes a great, positive and beneficial habit.

You are what you eat – so don't be fast, cheap, easy or fake!

Food allergies and intolerances

Just under 2% of people in the UK have a food allergy, but many more will have some form of food intolerance.

Food allergies:

- Symptoms come on within seconds or minutes of eating the food
- In extreme cases it can be life-threatening
- Even a tiny trace of the food can cause a reaction
- It is easily diagnosed with tests

A food allergy is a rapid and potentially serious response to a food by your immune system. It can trigger classic allergy symptoms such as a rash, wheezing and itching. The most common food allergies among adults are to fish and shellfish and nuts, including peanuts, walnuts, hazelnuts and brazil nuts. Children often have allergies to milk and eggs as well as to peanuts, other nuts and fish.

Food intolerances:

- Symptoms come on more slowly, are long-lasting, and mainly involve the digestive system
- It's never life-threatening
- A reasonable portion of food is usually needed to cause a reaction, although some people can be sensitive to small amounts
- You may crave the problem food
- It's difficult to diagnose as there are only a few reliable tests

Food intolerances are more common than food allergies. The symptoms of food intolerance tend to come on more slowly, often many hours after eating the problem food. Typical symptoms include bloating and stomach cramps. It's possible to be intolerant to several different foods; this can make it difficult to identify which foods are causing the problem. Food intolerances can also be difficult to tell apart from other digestive disorders that produce similar symptoms, such as inflammatory bowel disease, gastrointestinal obstructions or irritable bowel syndrome (IBS).

Lactose intolerance, sometimes known as dairy intolerance, occurs when your body can't digest lactose. Lactose is in milk and dairy products such as yoghurts and soft cheeses. The main symptoms are diarrhoea and stomach pain. In most cases, your GP can diagnose lactose intolerance by looking at your symptoms and medical history.

Sometimes it isn't clear which food is causing a problem. The only reliable way of identifying such a food intolerance is through an exclusion diet, where you cut out certain foods from your diet one at a time to see if there's an effect.

Coeliac disease is a common digestive condition where a person has an adverse reaction to gluten. However, coeliac disease is not an allergy or an intolerance to gluten. It is an autoimmune condition where the immune system mistakes substances found inside gluten as a threat to the body and attacks them. About 1% of the population in the UK have coeliac disease, though many of these aren't diagnosed.

Gluten is a protein found in wheat, rye and barley that damages the intestine of people with coeliac disease. Symptoms include diarrhoea, bloating and weight loss. Coeliac disease can be accurately diagnosed with a blood test and biopsy.

Treatments for food allergy and food intolerance

- In all cases, always read food labels carefully, and learn where your problem food may be used as an ingredient in other foods.

- In the case of a food allergy, you'll have to avoid the food you're allergic to. You may be able to eat the cooked versions without any problems, as can be the case with fruit or vegetable allergies.

- With lactose intolerance, you'll have to reduce the amount of dairy food that you eat.

- With other forms of food intolerance, you'll have to stop eating the food for a while, or possibly for life.

Case study
Losing 2½ stones for Kilimanjaro

It was just before Christmas 2012 and I was going with a group on a CYM trip to climb Kilimanjaro in mid-February 2013. One of the female members in the group had struggled with her weight for many years and when she signed up to the trip the previous spring it had helped motivate her to get fitter and lose quite a bit of weight. Things had been going quite well over the summer of 2012; she had lost some weight and was progressing with her exercise and fitness programme.

However, I had noticed she had stopped coming to some of the training activities; I hadn't seen her for a while from about mid-October and I was starting to get concerned. Kilimanjaro is an amazing trip and adventure but it is also a tough challenge and you want to be going into it with the confidence and belief you can successfully reach the summit. I contacted her around mid-December and she explained that she was struggling with various things; she had let her fitness and exercise regime falter and had been putting weight back on. She was losing her confidence and in turn her motivation.

I met with her and it was clear she had put a lot of weight back on and was not in a good place. Of course, I wanted her to reach the summit of Kilimanjaro and have a wonderful experience and feel the huge sense of achievement that brings, but to give her the best chance she had to get fitter and had to lose quite a lot of weight to help with that. So I suggested she follow a nutrition plan that I wrote for her and I agreed I would do some extra individual training with her to improve her fitness. She said she would give it a go and it was to start on 2nd January. This meant we had six weeks before we set off on the Kilimanjaro challenge.

Over Christmas I weighed myself and was slightly surprised to see that I had put on just over a stone in weight from the summer (when I did the 30 marathons in 30 days challenge – see the book *Motivation, Achievement & Challenges*) when I had to weigh myself regularly. Although I knew I had put on some weight and wasn't as fit as I had been it still surprised me and I thought perhaps I should try the same nutritional plan that I had suggested for this group member.

So on 2nd January we both began our new 'healthy eating for weight loss' programme – see the suggested nutrition plan below.

The first few days were a bit difficult but very soon it became a fairly easy habit and way of eating. Refusing sweets, cakes and chocolate became straightforward and sticking to the programme with only the very occasional 'treat' worked surprisingly easily. I never really felt hungry and my cravings for sugar decreased a lot. I also felt I had just as much energy as before and was able to do all my normal training. I met with the group member for additional training and got regular updates on her healthy eating programme; like me she found it fairly comfortable.

We continued to train and stick fairly closely to the eating plan and kept each other updated on how we were doing. 6 weeks later the results were in – in terms of weight I had lost exactly one stone (14lbs or 6.5kg) and she had lost one and a half stone (21lbs or 9.5kgs) so combined we had lost two and a half stone in 6 weeks by sticking to the nutritional plan! Furthermore, she was fitter and healthier, and her confidence and self-esteem had been boosted hugely. And she successfully made it to the top of Kilimanjaro – all 5,895 metres above sea-level – the highest free-standing mountain in the world!

Try it yourself!

Suggested Nutrition Plan

This was the plan we used and it was really about trying to reduce sugar intake as much as possible and limiting the carbohydrates to the low-calorie, slow-releasing energy food that is porridge. You could eat as many vegetables and salads as you wanted to, and quite a lot of lean protein. Combining these foods and factors it meant that overall calories were low but you felt fuller and the energy intake along with blood-sugar levels was much more consistent.

So the aim was to take out sugar, sweets, cakes, chocolate, breads, pastas, noodles, rice, potatoes etc., and processed foods. If you felt hungry then first call would be more vegetables and salad but if that didn't work then you could have more porridge. It is a sensible, consistent and sustainable nutrition and weight-loss plan and should help you maintain a healthier eating lifestyle going forward as you get used to eating more vegetables and salad and having porridge, and your cravings for high-sugar foods dramatically decrease.

Breakfast

- Bowl of plain porridge – with skimmed milk (plus honey or Demerara sugar or dried fruit pieces)

Lunch options

- Salad (lettuce, rocket, cucumber, tomatoes, peppers, radishes, pickled onions) plus smoked salmon and scrambled egg

- Tuna mayonnaise, cucumber, peppers, wholemeal pitta bread

- Salad plus chicken and hardboiled egg

- Omelette with peppers, onions, tomatoes and baked beans

Dinner options

- Chicken or turkey breast and vegetable stir fry (peppers, onions, bean shoots, courgettes, spinach, etc.)

- Fish and vegetables (broccoli, peas, carrots, sweetcorn, cabbage, French beans, etc.)

- Steak and vegetables

- Vegetarian options – pulses, beans, tofu, Quorn, etc.

Snacks if needed

- Additional salad and vegetables – as much as you like!

- Skimmed milk or skimmed milk milkshakes!

- Additional bowl of porridge if and when required

- Fruit – try to limit to 2 pieces per day

Summary and Moving Forward

The physical issues of being overweight

There is a wide range of potential health issues that will affect you physically by being overweight including a higher risk of type 2 diabetes, heart disease, strokes, some cancers and high blood pressure. Your sleep is more likely to be affected and if you are pregnant there may be increased risks to your baby. Understand the risks and use this as a motivator to get to a healthy weight for you.

The emotional issues of being overweight

Being overweight can cause mental and emotional health issues as for some people confidence and self-esteem will decrease and the risk of being depressed increases. They may become more isolated and withdrawn, become less social and take part in fewer activities. which will lead to a further lowering of confidence. They may face some forms of stigma and discrimination too, which further compound the issues.

Why are so many people overweight?

There are many factors as to why so many people are overweight and why this number is continuing to increase. Our modern twenty-first-century lifestyles mean we don't have to exercise and be physically active and we have a huge amount of choice regarding what we eat and drink – and we have easy access to this food and drink. Food retailers and manufacturers have laden so many products with addictive high-sugar content, and market unhealthy foods with so many offers and bargains.

However, at the end of the day you are responsible for the choices you make and what you eat and drink and how much physical activity you do, So take responsibility, make the changes, choose more carefully and healthily and you will notice a huge positive difference to your life.

How to lose weight effectively

The best way to lose weight effectively and to make it sustainable is to form good habits and make your lifestyle 'healthy' with a good balance of healthy eating and physical activity. The more it becomes a habit the easier it is to maintain and the more you practise, the easier it becomes a habit. Recognise and calculate the weight equation of calories in and calories out each day or each week.

Make sure you understand what your healthy weight is and how you can maintain a healthy lifestyle that works for you. Everyone is different, with different circumstances and practicalities, so do what works for you in a sensible way. Also try to ensure you have helpful, supportive and encouraging people around you who are a positive influence in your goals.

Healthy eating

The more healthily you eat (and drink) the better you will feel as you will have more energy, feel more positive, sleep better, lose weight if needed and you will be reducing your risk of a range of illnesses, diseases and other health issues. There are so many benefits of healthy eating and you can be fully responsible for what you eat and the good habits you can adopt.

Take more time to think about how you can eat more healthily, by planning and preparing your meals, buying the right foods, avoiding temptations, enjoying the healthy foods, eating at the right times, having a good balance and controlling your portion sizes.

Understanding foods

Probably the best way to eat healthily is to have a good understanding of foods – what is in them, and what the benefits and dangers are. The more knowledge you have the better informed you will be and the more motivated to make the healthier choices.

Understanding labels is important, so make it a habit to check what is in the food you buy and consume. Don't be misled or tempted by the marketing, promotions and offers of the unhealthy, sugar-rich, high-calorie products, be aware of what drinks contain as well as foods and don't forget the benefits of water.

Other factors

If you have children try to educate them about food and the health risks of being overweight; encourage them to eat healthily and try to set a good example. Seek out friends who will be encouraging and supportive with the goals you have to eat better and exercise more.

Try to reduce or cut out sugar and eat a lot more vegetables and salad, perhaps growing and eating your own produce. See 'treats' as something you have very occasionally for special occasions rather than as a daily occurrence and if you are comfort eating try to address the underlying issues that are likely to be around self-esteem, anxiety, stress or depression.

Be healthier, happier and live longer!

You really are what you eat and if you eat healthily then you will be healthier. You will also feel happier and much more likely to live longer. The effort in losing weight, being more active and eating more healthily is worth the reward.

It can be difficult for many reasons, but if you understand them then address those reasons and you will be able to make a big difference to your life. Your confidence and self-esteem will increase, you will have more energy, you will sleep better and be more positive. You will do more with your life and be a great example and inspiration to others too.

Go for it and stick with it and you will see and feel the results – and it will become easier. Those previous hard choices will become easier and the previous easy choices will become less attractive. You will be so pleased with your new healthier lifestyle and all the benefits it brings with it!

The CYM Weight Loss Challenge

A great way to lose weight, eat more healthily, feel great yourself and help our charity at the same time is to take part in the CYM Weight Loss challenge!

You can do this at any time – it is essentially a 4-week healthy eating challenge, which if done right, will certainly mean you will lose weight if you are currently overweight. Plus you can ask people to sponsor you for this challenge, which not only raises money for the charity but will give you an additional motivational factor (hopefully!).

If you email info@climbyourmountain.org we will send you more details of the challenge and how best to raise sponsorship, plus we will help support you and motivate you for the 4 weeks of the challenge.

So if you would like to help us and do something really beneficial for yourself at the same time then please get in touch and start the weight loss challenge. I look forward to hearing from you!

About the
'Climb Your Mountain' Charity

The Climb Your Mountain (CYM) charity was set up in 2008 by Charlie Wardle with the aim of helping anyone who felt they had their own personal mountain to climb in life. CYM offers advice, support, information, education, activities and opportunities for people to help themselves improve their health and happiness and effectively climb their own personal mountain.

Everyone will go through difficult times in life which may include work issues, relationship problems, financial pressures, health concerns, low confidence, anxiety, depression, social isolation, bereavement, etc., and Climb Your Mountain (CYM) offers a range of opportunities for people to help them through these difficult times in a number of ways.

CYM Health offers a range of free practical, easy-to-read, informative self-help books, as well as free online video workshops on the same topics for people to view and benefit from. Charlie Wardle also delivers talks, seminars, courses and workshops to the general public and to companies on a range of health and wellbeing topics.

To fund the charity and be able to offer all the free CYM Health services, the CYM Challenges division offers a range of fantastic trips and challenges across the UK and also some overseas trips. Anyone can participate in these great-value trips and challenges and have an amazing experience whilst also helping to support and fund the charity.

To find out more about the 'Climb Your Mountain' charity:

Website www.climbyourmountain.org

Email info@climbyourmountain.org

We rely heavily for funding on people making donations and raising money from taking part in trips and challenges. If you can help by making a donation please go to

www.justgiving.com/climbym

or get in touch and take part in a trip or challenge with us!

You can also TEXT a £5 donation to the charity

TEXT: BOOK32£5

To: 70070

Or an online donation via:

www.justgiving.com/healthbooks

THANK YOU!